Surgical Nursing
A Concise Nursing Text

Maureen Wilson BA SRN RNT
Lecturer in Nursing Studies
University of Surrey

Eleventh Edition

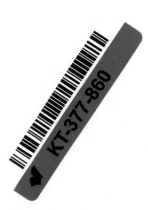

Baillière Tindall London Philadelphia Toronto
Sydney Tokyo

Baillière Tindall   24-28 Oval Road
W. B. Saunders   London NW1 7DX

The Curtis Center, Independence
Square West, Philadelphia, PA
19106-3399, USA

55 Horner Avenue
Toronto, Ontario M8Z 4X6, Canada

Harcourt Brace Jovanovich Group
(Australia) Pty Ltd.,
30-52 Smidmore St, Marrickville,
NSW 2204, Australia

Harcourt Brace Jovanovich (Japan) Inc.
Ichibancho Central Building, 22—1 Ichibancho
Chiyoda-ku, Tokyo 102, Japan

This book is printed on acid-free paper ∞

First published 1938
Tenth edition 1979
Eleventh edition 1985
Fourth printing 1992

Sinhala edition (Sri Lanka Government)
Spanish translation, ninth edition (CECSA, Mexico)
Turkish edition (Turkish Government)
Portuguese translation, ninth edition (Publicações Europa-America,
Portugal)
Dutch translation, ninth edition (Stafleu, The Netherlands)

Published in an English Language Book Society edition

Typeset by Cotswold Typesetting Ltd, Cheltenham
Printed in England by Clays Ltd, St Ives plc

British Library Cataloguing in Publication Data
Wilson, Maureen
  Surgical nursing.—11th ed.—(Nurses' aids series)
  1. Surgical nursing
  I. Title II. Series
  610.73'677   RD99
ISBN 0 7020 1061-8

Contents

Foreword

This new edition has been completely rewritten in order that it may more effectively assist nurses to plan care based upon the identified needs of individual patients. This has been achieved by using a systematic, problem-orientated approach to the care of the surgical patient.

Nurses now recognize their responsibility and accountability for planning meaningful, safe care based upon the four key stages of the 'nursing process': **assessment** of the patient and the identification of needs or problems, **planning** for the short and long term after specifying the desired outcome of care, **implementation** of the planned care, and **evaluation** to monitor achievement of the goals.

Many different models of care have been described, such as 'activities of living' (Roper, Logan and Tierney, 1980), 'self care' (Orem, 1971) and 'stress adaptation' (Saxton and Hyland, 1979); the author has chosen to discuss principles of care and not to concentrate on any one model, allowing readers to apply the principles of care to their own model of choice. The author and the publishers have decided to use this approach because of the gradual transformation in the system of care that has taken place within the last two decades; it is now based upon a nursing model rather than a medical model.

In 1976 the World Health Organization introduced its 'Medium-Term Programme in Nursing and Midwifery' into Europe. One of its components was the introduction of the nursing process into named European countries, one of them being the United Kingdom. This was carried out using a system of Type 1 and Type 2 centres, Link nurses from the Regions and designated nursing process development/advisory posts within the Health Authorities. In 1979 the General Nursing Council issued their Statement of Educational Policy (77/19/A), in which they stated, 'the concept of the nursing process provides a unifying thread for the study of patient care and a helpful framework for nursing practice'.

Using the nursing process approach has resulted in a wide

range of subjective observations, such as statements that it improves the standard of care of some patients and increases job satisfaction for staff. However, there is a need for further research to be carried out into the effectiveness of the nursing process, as there have been few attempts to do this within the field of surgical nursing. Sellick and Russell (1983) found higher levels of patient and staff satisfaction in acute medical and surgical wards when primary nursing was introduced, but little other evidence has been produced.

This new edition admirably illustrates this method of planning care for patients who require the aid of professionals to assist them to overcome the problems that they have encountered. It will be of great assistance to both learners and trained staff in learning to implement this systematic, problem-orientated method of caring for surgical patients.

E. J. Fish
August 1984

1
Surgical Nursing

It is the aim of this book to structure nursing care according to perceived need. Every nurse formulates an individual model of care according to the manner in which she conceptualizes the nurse–patient relationship, but it is generally acknowledged that a nurse has a responsibility to assist, to comfort and to support when these activities are appropriate, and to advise and teach in order that a patient may preserve his integrity and be in possession of sufficient information to make informed decisions.

- A process of nursing constructs care logically and systematically, in order that identified needs are met.
- A need will become a problem if it is not met.
- A nursing care plan is designed to meet specific individual needs and by definition can never be routine care.
- Implicit in a plan of care for a patient who will undergo surgery is that the nurse is responsible for the patient's safety and the preservation of his integrity when he is unable to control his own environment, for example, when he is affected by premedication, anaesthesia and postoperative analgesia.
- Any 'model of care' may be implemented, for all models are concerned with the patient's ability to adapt his normal activities to altered circumstances and to process along a continuum from dependence to independence.
- A plan of care is positively evaluated by the extent to which objectives are achieved.
- Documentation—prescriptions and definitions of care—is the foundation on which professional responsibility and public accountability are based.
- Care plans are nursing tools and should be the basis for scientific practice. They are a source for replicating and validating existing nursing theory, rejecting outdated practice and generating new nursing knowledge.

Table 1. Plan of care

Need	Related nursing activity (page reference)
On admission	
Orientation to ward:	3
Geography	3
People	3
Information	3
Preparation for surgery	
Immediate	
Knowledge	4
Confidence	4
Continuing	
Social—relatives	5
Psychological—preparation	6
Physical—Premedication and preparation—	6
safety	7
On return from theatre	
Airway	9
Vital signs	12
Relief of pain/discomfort	14
Fluid intake/urine output	15
Blood transfusion	18
Continuing care	
Nutrition	19
Bowel activity	21
Mobility	21
Hygiene	22
Wound care	
Drainage	24
Closure	26
Removal of sutures	28
Conditions for wound healing	29
Nutritional status	30
Defence mechanisms	30
Circulatory status	31
Prevention of wound infection	32
Safe environment	32
Wound management—asepsis	35
Sterility of equipment etc.	36
Disinfectants and antiseptics	37

Table 1. Plan of care—*continued*

Need	Related nursing activity (page reference)
Nursing in isolation	
Knowledge/information	39
Protection	39
Support—patient and relatives	40
Preparation for discharge	
Adequate information	42
Support	42
Services	42
Time for mental preparation	42
Advice—social services	44

ON ADMISSION

People enter hospital with needs which will vary according to their past experiences and knowledge of the events to follow. There will be apprehension and sometimes fear and it is therefore essential that the first impressions are positive. Many hospitals engage non-nursing staff to escort patients to their designated wards in a friendly, informal manner.

Identification of needs
- Orientation to the ward.

Related nursing activities
- Admission. This should be as unbureaucratic as possible, friendly and welcoming; the unexpected patient for whom no provision has been made should be kept unaware of this fact as far as possible.
- The geography of the ward. The vital aspects, for example the disposition of lavatories, bathrooms and fire exits, should be introduced immediately, but the patient should not be flooded with a mass of information, which he will not be able to assimilate all at once.
- Introduction to fellow patients. This initial introduction should be carried out formally and the patients allowed to determine the social level at which they wish to interact.
- Detailed information. Any written information which may

have been sent to the patient before his admission should be reinforced, where necessary, with further details, for example, the ward telephone number, any restrictions on visiting hours and the age group of those visiting, the distinction between uniforms, and who will best be able to meet any need for further specific help and information.

- Valuables. If possible, a facility for locking away personal valuables should be made available.
- Ward 'milestones'. Information about the times at which meals are usually served and tea and coffee are available is an important early essential.
- Timetable of events. If possible the time at which the doctor will visit the patient and any other investigations which are planned, together with the preparation necessary, should be given; thereafter, the patient can be allowed to adjust to his environment as he wishes.

Ideally this early introduction to the ward should be carried out by the nurse who will be responsible for making a nursing care assessment and supporting the patient throughout the ensuing days.

PREPARATION FOR SURGERY

Identification of needs
- Knowledge of events, to enable the patient to cooperate in all preparations which will promote an uncomplicated recovery.
- Confidence in those responsible for his care, that his integrity and safety will be maintained at all times.

Related nursing activities
Social assessment. Any information which is directly relevant to the surgical outcome should be sought; for example, after a lower limb amputation will the patient need to climb stairs at home? Some information may not appear to be directly relevant, but may affect the patient's ability to respond to, for instance, marital problems or difficulties over children's schooling; information such as this must be respected and constructive efforts made, where appropriate, to locate a supporting agency who may be able to help. Financial and employment difficulties may

become an overwhelming worry and consequently dissipate energies which are needed to cope with postoperative recovery.

Psychological assessment. It is rarely possible to gain insight into the patient's adjustment in the limited time available, but it is important to ascertain how much he understands about his condition and what is to happen to him and to make some assessment of mental readiness. It will be difficult to decide if an aggressive or irritable response is a sign of underlying tension, but these signs may help the nurse to match her care more nearly to the needs of the patient.

Physical assessment. 'Base-line' observations will be used to assess immediate and continuing postoperative responses. These should include temperature, pulse and respiratory rate, blood pressure and weight recordings, together with urinalysis. They should be charted and included on those charts relevant for operating theatre use. Any abnormalities should be reported. Any specimens, such as urine and sputum, together with swabs from orifices should be obtained, correctly labelled and despatched for appropriate investigations. From the patient's perspective there are no 'routine' investigations and each specimen should be obtained only after the patient has been given clear and specific information. Information and restrictions related to investigations must be accurate and appear logical to the patient. Smoking restrictions should be explained with care and consideration.

The doctor may seek assistance when obtaining blood samples for haemoglobin estimation, grouping and cross-matching. These are aseptic techniques and specimens should be handled with care (as should any other secretions).

Preoperative nursing care

Social care

Relatives and friends must be informed of the nature of the operation, the approximate time that it will be carried out and when it will be possible to telephone for news concerning the patient's immediate postoperative condition; they should also be told of the earliest occasion when a visit to the patient can be permitted.

Psychological care

Information about the specific timing of events, in other words the place on the theatre list and the timing of the premedication, may reduce anxiety.

Physical care

Skin preparations. A bath is usually desirable and antiseptic solutions may be added. Nails must be clean and varnish-free. The umbilicus is frequently a neglected area. If the patient is aware of these normal hygiene requirements he can take the major responsibility for this preparation.

The surgeon may require the skin in the area of the operation to be free of hair, but care must be taken to prevent damage to the skin; this is usually easier with a wet shave than with a dry one.

A theatre gown will be worn by the patient and the bed to which he returns must be clean and freshly made.

Surgical stockings which apply external pressure to the superficial veins of the lower limbs may be ordered by the surgeon. The reason for their use should be explained: they may inhibit the formation of deep vein thrombosis by preventing stasis in the superficial veins of the lower limbs.

Bowel preparation. It is usually required that the patient should have an empty rectum. Aperients may have been prescribed; glycerol suppositories or a small disposable enema may be administered. The patient should be consulted about his normal bowel activity.

Food and fluid restriction. Food and fluids will be restricted for at least six hours before the premedication is due, and it should be stressed that 'nil by mouth' includes both eating and drinking. A bath, taken when meals are being served in the ward, may divert attention from the desire to eat, and particularly to drink, when others are enjoying their breakfast or lunch.

Drugs. Some drugs must be continued even when food and fluids are restricted; the drug-prescription chart should be checked on the routine medicine rounds.

Administration of a premedication
A combination of a drug which will sedate with a drug which will reduce secretions is usually given one hour before the operation or as ordered. Two examples, both given by intramuscular injection, are: (a) papaveretum 20 mg (a narcotic analgesic) with hyoscine hydrobromide 0.4 mg (400 µg) (an antisialogogue) and (b) pethidine 100 mg with atropine 0.6 mg (600 µg); these doses may be reduced according to the age and the weight of the patient. An additional effect of the premedication is to enhance the effect of subsequent anaesthesia. Premedication may be prescribed orally, for example lorazepam 2 mg, which induces light sedation; it may be preceded by a similar dose the previous night. If oral premedication is prescribed, a minimal amount of water, sufficient to swallow the tablets, is offered.

Guidelines must be followed prior to administration. If there is a checklist to be completed, it must be remembered that the patient is more important than the checklist. Such a list will contain details of the patient's age and any relevant identifying number to be checked against an identification label. It should be established that a formal consent to the operative procedure, signed by the patient and witnessed by a doctor after discussion, is in existence. A check should be made on whether dentures and other prostheses have been removed; safe custody of jewellery is to be ensured. A hearing aid should never be removed until after the patient has been anaesthetized, when it should be clearly labelled and deposited in a safe place. Immediately after the operation it should be reinserted while the patient is still in the recovery area. Finally, before the premedication is given the patient must be asked to empty his bladder. The effects of the premedication should be carefully explained: he will feel rather sleepy and his mouth will feel very dry.

Controlled drugs should be administered according to hospital guidelines and the statutory requirements of the Misuse of Drugs Act (1971).

The patient's safety. After the premedication has been given the safety of the patient is entirely the responsibility of the nurse. He must be asked not to attempt to get out of bed but assured that assistance is readily available; a bell to summon assistance must be within reach. It is safer for the patient not to be screened off and the door to a single room should remain open.

All relevant documents—notes, X-rays, and current investigation results, such as haemoglobin measurements and ECG—should be gathered together.

The nurse who has been responsible for the preparation of the patient should escort him to the operating theatre and remain with him until anaesthesia is induced, assisting the anaesthetist as required.

Anaesthesia

Local anaesthesia (loss of sensation) may be induced by blocking conduction along nerve fibres, for example by:

a topical application to mucous membranes
b infiltration
c regional nerve block
d epidural and caudal block.

General anaesthetics act by depressing the central nervous system.

Stages of general anaesthesia

Stage 1   Analgesia: lasts until the patient is unconscious.
Stage 2   Delirium: lasts from the onset of unconsciousness until automatic regular breathing begins. At this stage the patient sometimes holds his breath and struggles.
Stage 3   Surgical anaesthesia: lasts from the onset of automatic breathing until the respiratory centre is paralysed.
Stage 4   Overdosage: the short interval between cessation of breathing and death if untreated.

General anaesthesia may be administered by intravenous injection alone, for induction and short surgical procedures, or by inhalation of gases or volatile liquids, for induction and maintenance of anaesthesia. Muscle relaxants block neuromuscular transmission, permitting a light level of anaesthesia with adequate muscle relaxation.

Postoperative respiratory depression may be reversed by the administration of naloxone hydrochloride (Narcan).

ON RETURN FROM THE OPERATING THEATRE

The ultimate aim of nursing care is to facilitate recovery without complications. Care must be systematically planned to meet nursing goals related to patient needs. A plan of care should maintain continuity from a state of patient dependency immediately after the operation to one of independence and eventual self-care, if this ultimate desirable state is attainable.

Identification of needs

While the patient is dependent, that is, he has not recovered completely from the effects of the anaesthetic and is unable to carry out those physical activities which are essential for his well-being, it is the responsibility of the nurse to make a comprehensive assessment, to enable her to:

- Maintain an airway
- Monitor vital signs
- Alleviate pain and discomfort
- Monitor fluid intake/output
- Communicate an effective account of his condition.

Related nursing activities

It is common practice for patients to be nursed in a recovery area close to the operating theatre, until it is considered safe to proceed to the ward. This decision is the responsibility of the anaesthetist.

Assessment begins immediately the patient has been assigned to the receiving nurse's care, but this will not be possible until she is in possession of written information as follows:

- The nature of the operation which has been performed
- Any specific instructions regarding immediate care requested by the surgeon or anaesthetist
- A charted account of postoperative recovery
- Any analgesia which has been administered in the recovery area and the time it was given.

Superficial observation at this stage will reveal:

- The patient's respiratory activity
- His general appearance, and the colour of his face and extremities
- Whether he feels cold or is sweating excessively
- Whether he is restless, disorientated or in pain
- The presence of an intravenous infusion and drainage tubes
- The incision and presence of dressings.

Maintenance of airway adequacy

This is necessary to prevent respiratory obstruction and to avoid an aspiration pneumonia.

Until the patient has regained consciousness and a cough reflex is present, he should not be left unattended. Positioning should ideally be semi-prone (Figure 1). This is not always possible after some types of surgery, such as hip replacement operations; if the semi-prone position is not possible, the head should be positioned to prevent the tongue falling back and obstructing the oropharynx (Figure 2). Forward pressure exerted with the fingers at the angle of the jaw or below the chin will prevent this happening.

It is essential that the foot of the bed can be elevated, enabling the head to be tipped. Suction apparatus should be available to remove excess secretions from the airway, and the possibility that the patient might vomit should be uppermost in the nurse's mind, especially if the preparation for surgery was of an emergency nature or the effects of the anaesthesia have not been fully reversed. Vomit may be aspirated (sucked) into the respiratory tract and cause an aspiration pneumonia; this is a potentially serious condition and a considerable setback to ultimate, uneventful, uncomplicated recovery.

As soon as the patient is responsive, he must be encouraged to move freely (as far as any restricting drainage tubes, splints, dressings and so on allow) and to carry out lung expansion exercises practised prior to the operation. It is especially difficult to breathe deeply and expand the lungs fully when pain is present, but it is essential to persist with these exercises to prevent consolidation of secretions at the bases of the lungs. It is sometimes helpful to 'splint' the painful part—supporting the abdomen by holding a firm pillow against the abdominal wall—but pain

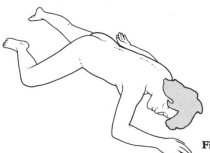

Figure 1. The semi-prone position.

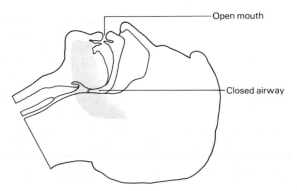

Figure 2a. The open mouth allows the tongue to fall back and block the airway.

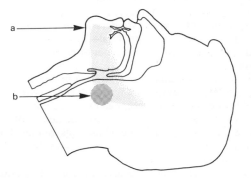

Figure 2b. Gentle pressure exerted by the fingertips in the direction indicated (a) below the chin, closing the mouth, or (b) at the 'angle of the jaw' will maintain a clear airway.

should of course be relieved before any attempt is made to gain the patient's cooperation in carrying out essential but uncomfortable exercises. The administration of narcotics will be determined by normal respiratory rate. A sputum container should be within easy reach, together with paper tissues and a mouthwash solution.

Oxygen may be prescribed (on the instructions of the anaesthetist) to relieve hypoxia. It is possible to deliver oxygen at specific concentrations—for example, a venturi mask mixes oxygen with air and can control oxygen concentrations between 24% and 40%. The exact requirement should be clearly specified. Some patients with chronic obstructive airways disease rely on low oxygen concentrations for their respiratory drive and in such cases the correct concentration is an important factor. This is because, whereas normally a rise in carbon dioxide concentration causes an increase in respiration, the respiratory centre in these patients has become conditioned to a higher concentration of carbon dioxide by the decreased oxygen intake. They therefore rely on a decreased oxygen concentration in the blood to stimulate respiration. A sudden large increase in the oxygen concentration could cause such patients to stop breathing.

Masks are often uncomfortable (although adjustable to suit each face) and provoke anxiety; the patient must be assured of the safety of the procedure, and the reasons for his need for oxygen should be clearly explained. Safety precautions regarding the presence of oxygen cylinders at the bedside or oxygen delivery through wall fitments should be followed according to hospital guidelines. Smoking must not be permitted in the vicinity of oxygen.

Arterial blood specimens may be taken for assessment of blood gases. For this purpose, a syringe (primed with heparin) is required by the doctor; the specimen must be immediately taken for analysis and not allowed to wait for the next routine collection. The site from which the blood was obtained requires continuous pressure to prevent haematoma formation, and should be checked subsequently.

Check chest X-rays may be ordered; these investigations must be preceded by careful explanation of their necessity.

Continuing respiratory well-being and gradually increasing mobility are interdependent; however, they cannot be achieved until an adequate circulatory response has been established.

Monitoring vital signs—pulse, blood pressure and temperature

Identification of needs

The patient needs a stable blood pressure and pulse rate which compare favourably with recordings made before the operation.

Related nursing activities

Assessment of pulse and blood pressure recordings. A rising pulse rate and a falling systolic blood pressure may indicate a fall in circulating blood volume as a result of bleeding. Drainage tubing and the wound site should be observed for external signs of bleeding and the findings reported immediately. The patient may also be restless or confused, and the skin may feel cold and clammy. Elevating the foot of the bed, when appropriate, may raise the systolic pressure in the short term, but alternative measures must be considered. Oxygen should be administered via a face mask until a medical reassessment has been made.

The blood pressure will remain low if bleeding is present and not treated; the patient may need to return to the operating theatre for investigation and possible religation of bleeding vessels.

Sufficient fluid must be given intravenously to replace blood lost while on the theatre table. Replacement with crystalloid preparations alone will not increase the blood pressure if the circulating blood volume is grossly depleted (see p. 15).

If the patient is in pain the blood pressure may remain low, and the continuing effect of the anaesthetics used may reduce blood pressure.

As the pulse rate and blood pressure stabilize recordings may be carried out at decreasing intervals until ultimately they are no longer necessary.

Temperature. This will not be of immediate concern and a recording every four hours is usually adequate. However, an increase in the temperature suggests the presence of infection. An early rise may be the first sign of a chest infection, but specimens of both sputum and urine should be obtained for culture of any organisms present and the sensitivity determined. Antimicrobial drugs will be given as prescribed.

Charting of observations. This is an important responsibility, but is a reliable nursing tool only if the recordings are related to the general appearance of the patient, the medications he is being prescribed and the patient's own interpretation of his symptoms.

Alleviation of pain and discomfort

Identification of needs

It is within the experience of most nurses that the alleviation of pain is the key to an uncomplicated recovery after surgery. Early mobility becomes a realistic goal, breathing exercises are easier to accomplish and recovery is generally quicker. It is also recognized that when a truthful estimate of the extent of the discomfort and the length of time it can be expected to last is offered, together with the information that relief is always available, anxiety tends to be reduced, thus permitting the patient to maintain his dignity and his personal integrity.

Related nursing activities

Assessment of pain. Many patients are stoical regarding personal discomfort. If not articulated, pain may be apparent from systemic signs: a reduced systolic blood pressure and raised pulse rate (see previous observations), a tense, anxious expression, pallor and sweating; the patient may adopt a rigid position and his breathing may be shallow in an attempt to 'splint' the surgical incision by reducing respiratory movement.

Analgesia. Analgesic drugs are often prescribed according to the patient's age and body weight; a prescription of 10–20 mg of papaveretum gives the nurse some degree of decision-making freedom. Antiemetics in the phenothiazine group, often prescribed simultaneously, should be considered for their sedative effect even if the patient is not nauseated or vomiting. Pain should be anticipated and analgesia administered accordingly, rather than allowing the patient's threshold of pain to be breached. Narcotic drugs will not begin to be effective until about half an hour after administration intramuscularly.

The immediate pain of a surgical incision usually gives way to a feeling of soreness at the site; this may be relieved by analgesia of the non-narcotic type; for example, paracetamol 0.5–1.0 g orally every four to six hours, or aspirin 300–600 mg, orally every four to six hours (note that aspirin is contraindicated when anticoagulant therapy is concurrent or in the presence of gastrointestinal disorders).

Pain not normally associated with the operation performed should be reported; for example calf pain, which may be associated with deep vein thrombosis, pleural pain, which may be embolic in origin, and pain at the site of an intravenous infusion.

Alternative sources of pain relief. These include altering the position of limbs, relieving pressure, providing sheepskins or the warmth of a soft blanket (a cuddly!) directly next to the skin; extra pillows tucked well down behind the neck will often be effective. A warm drink, the ubiquitous cup of tea and, most particularly, quiet conversation and the ability to listen in the small (but long) hours are invaluable nursing aids to pain relief.

Private worries about employment, finances, children's well-being, and fears about the operation can reduce the threshold for pain.

Fluid balance

Homeostasis must be maintained after any surgical procedure and it is often the case that oral fluids will be restricted until normal gut function is present (indicated by the return of bowel sounds—see p. 107) and fluids can be assimilated; at the same time, stomach contents may be aspirated. The patient may therefore be deficient in both water and electrolytes, and these will need to be replaced by intravenous infusion.

Intravenous infusion

Identification of needs
- Safety in respect of (a) equipment used, (b) fluids infused and (c) local care at the site of infusion
- Comfort: for example, movement may be restricted
- Knowledge about the equipment: to enable the patient to contribute to his own care

Related nursing activities
- When the infusion is commenced the equipment must remain uncontaminated whilst the giving set is assembled, the infusion fluid is run through the tubing and the tubing is connected to the intravenous cannula.
- The doctor may require assistance whilst he is cannulating the vein; the bed linen must be protected and kept clean and dry.

- The patient must be prepared for the procedure, by careful explanation, as it proceeds.
- The site to be cannulated (Figure 3) should be shaved if necessary and cleaned with an antiseptic solution.
- Before connecting the giving set to the cannula the tubing must be free of any air bubbles.
- The cannula should be adequately strapped (any allergy to strapping materials having been noted), and splinted only if necessary, i.e. if the cannula has been inserted at the antecubital fossa or at the wrist. A cannula inserted into a vein in the forearm is usually splinted by the underlying bone and does not normally need to be further restricted.
- Before the patient is left resting comfortably, the flow rate of the infusion should be calculated according to the amount

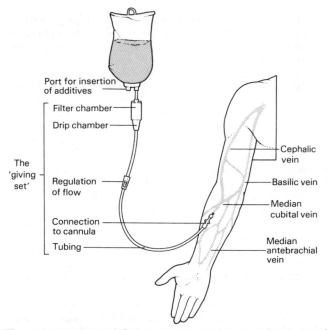

Figure 3. Intravenous infusion equipment and the superficial veins of the forearm that may be cannulated.

prescribed and the number of hours over which it is to be infused. To calculate flow rate in drops per minute the total volume of fluid to be infused, multiplied by the number of drops per millilitre delivered by the giving set (usually 15 drops per millilitre for crystalloids and 12 drops per millilitre for colloids), is divided by the time in minutes over which it is to be infused, thus:

$$\frac{\text{Volume of fluid (ml)} \times \text{drops per ml}}{\text{Time (hours)} \times 60}$$

For example, to give one litre of normal saline over eight hours using a giving set which delivers 15 drops per millilitre, the flow rate required is:

$$\frac{1000 \text{ ml} \times 15 \text{ drops/ml}}{8 \text{ h} \times 60 \text{ min}} = 31 \text{ drops per minute}$$

- Any additive, for example potassium, if not added to the infusion fluid under controlled conditions by the pharmacy, must be added by the nurse after checking, according to hospital policy, and the bag clearly labelled.
- A fluid chart should be completed, stating the nature of the infusion and the time at which the next unit is to be commenced.
- The patient must be left comfortable and properly clothed (pyjama jacket on); items which he may need should be placed on the appropriate side of the bed, within his reach.
- The site should regularly be checked for signs of inflammation or extravasation.
- Drugs such as antimicrobials can be administered as a bolus, either via the cannula, when an access port is present for this purpose, or into the rubber bung of the giving set. They may also be inserted as an additive into the infusion solution; hospital guidelines must be observed (some hospitals restrict the drugs which can be administered by nursing staff). There are also precautions to be taken regarding protective clothing to be worn when giving drugs used in cytotoxic therapy.
- The first dose, and preferably the second one, is usually given by a doctor. A check should also be made for drug incompatibility: some drugs when added to a solution will alter its pH, others become ineffective when infused over time, whilst

some are ineffective when exposed to light. Pharmacy advice is invaluable when any doubt exists.

- Hands must be clean and dry.
- The patient must be observed for reactions (see below).
- A cannula may be inserted, via a deep vein such as the right internal jugular or subclavian vein, into the right atrium for an accurate assessment of the circulating blood volume. The cannula is attached via a three-way tap to a manometer and a giving set. The tap controls the entry of infusion fluid to the manometer and the patient. When the zero point on the manometer is level with the manubrio-sternal angle, the pressure recorded by the manometer will vary from —5 to +5 cm of water (—500 to +500 Pa). It is any variation in the pressure which is significant, so the patient should be similarly positioned for each recording. This access should not be considered for drug administration. The position of this cannula is always checked by X-ray immediately after its insertion. Careful observation must be made of the patient's pulse, blood pressure and respiratory rate. Septicaemia should be suspected if an elevated temperature persists.

Blood transfusion

- The same precautions must be taken as for infusion (above); in addition, hospitals have specific guidelines for the administration of blood transfusions, which must be followed meticulously.
- Rigorous checking of the patient's blood group against the unit to be transfused, together with the expiry date of the blood, must be carried out by those authorized to do so.
- Close and regular observation of the patient's pulse rate, blood pressure and temperature must be made in order to detect any allergic reaction to the blood transfusion. Any of the following signs and symptoms should be reported immediately and the transfusion stopped:
  a Rise in temperature
  b Increased pulse or respiratory rate
  c Change in blood pressure
  d Dyspnoea (pleural oedema)
  e Any low back or loin pain
  f Any rash or facial swelling

An antihistamine drug will be given intravenously by the doctor, together with hydrocortisone and a diuretic such as frusemide. The remaining blood, together with all equipment, will be returned to the haematology department for further investigations.

Continuing care

When it is considered that the patient is able to absorb via the gastrointestinal tract, fluids will be offered orally, in slowly increasing amounts, until eventually he is able to take unrestricted fluids and is also able to eat. Fluid intake must be balanced against output after most surgical procedures. There are exceptions, such as some cardiac surgery, where intake is restricted and output is greater. Output factors to be considered are drainage (considered later in this chapter under 'Wounds') and urine production.

Parenteral nutrition

If for some reason the patient is unable to absorb via the gastrointestinal tract (for instance, if a fistula is present), total parenteral nutrition will be instituted. For this purpose a central vein, usually the subclavian, will be cannulated. The patient's individual nutritional needs can be met by concentrated amino acid, lipid and carbohydrate products; vitamins can also be added. Asepsis is essential throughout any procedure connected with the feeding regimen and the dangers associated with septicaemia must always be a serious consideration when any manoeuvre is carried out.

The subclavian cannulation is especially difficult for the patient to come to terms with and every effort must be made to reassure him of his safety and provide for his comfort.

Urine production

After surgical procedures this may decrease initially but should return to normal (1 ml/min) within 24 hours. There may be difficulty with micturition for various reasons:
- Physiological—after surgical handling in the pelvic region.
- Psychological—inability to use a urinal in bed or a commode in the ward area.

Related nursing activities

- If the bladder is palpable and the patient is unable to pass urine despite the usual remedies—privacy, running taps and so on—efforts should be made to ascertain the cause and to deal with it as appropriate.
- Catheterization is a last resort: urinary tract infection after this procedure is a well-recognized hazard. However, if a catheter is to be inserted, strict aseptic precautions must be observed. The meatus must be kept clean and the drainage bag emptied, with due regard to the risk of introducing pathogens into the urinary tract.
- The presence of a urinary catheter may be distressing to the patient and the preservation of his dignity must be observed on all occasions involving catheter care.
- Measurement and urinalysis should be charted and any abnormalities should be reported.

Continuing care

Identification of needs

- Adequate nutritional status
- Increasing mobility—to reduce risk of circulatory complications
- Hygiene—to prevent infection

Related nursing activities

Nutritional status
Improved technology in the hospital system often means that nurses are no longer concerned with either preparing or serving meals to patients: nevertheless the patient's nutritional well-being is a prime responsibility. The nurse must assist the patient who has no restrictions on his diet to choose appropriately and be able to suggest alternatives which will satisfy the requirements for a balanced diet and meet the calorific (energy) needs of a patient recovering after surgery. She is also responsible for ensuring that the meal chosen has been eaten and should be able to offer alternatives, for example meat extracts, proprietary preparations such as Complan and flavoured milk products. Relatives are sensitive to the patient's food preferences and may be able to bring in items which will tempt a jaded appetite. This

applies especially to ethnic minorities, for whom food in hospitals may be a special difficulty, although many hospital kitchens now cater for most minority groups.

- After a period when diet has been restricted to fluids-only, it is common to reintroduce solid food with a light diet, for instance clear soups and milk puddings, and gradually increase this, together with fruit juices, fresh fruit and bran added to cereal in order to increase the dietary fibre content of the meals with a view to promoting normal bowel activity.
- Bowel activity after surgery. It is often necessary to give suppositories (glycerine) to initiate bowel action; thereafter a normal diet with extra dietary fibre should maintain this activity. A mild aperient such as Dorbanex 10 ml at night, may be prescribed until the patient has returned to a relatively normal lifestyle, his own home surroundings and exercise pattern.

Mobility
This must be increased gently, as the patient's condition allows. Mobility is important for a number of reasons:
- It promotes venous return from the lower limbs, thus preventing venous stasis and deep vein thrombosis.
- It promotes maximum lung expansion, which may not always be attainable whilst in bed, despite the use of bed aids and the patient's cooperation.
- It prevents undue pressure on vulnerable areas, which could cause skin breakdown, the development of pressure sores and consequently delay recovery.

Related nursing activities. The patient must be confident in his ability to get out of bed safely; the bed area must be properly organized, a chair of the appropriate height made available and unnecessary furniture cleared away. His slippers and dressing gown should be prepared and any attached drainage tubes taken to the correct side of the bed before the move is undertaken. Explicit directions must be given regarding what the patient has to do and every effort made to allow him to do as much as he wishes to do for himself; analgesia may be necessary before the activity is considered. A clear undertaking should be given that he will be able to get back when he is ready, and a means of summoning assistance must be available to him. He must be warm and protected from draught and excessive movement around him in the ward. A balance between the time spent in bed and up in a chair should be achieved.

Signs of a possible venous thrombosis must be recognized; there may be a rise in the pulse rate, with elevated temperature, and calf tenderness and swelling with a positive Homans' sign. Heparin may be commenced intravenously to prevent further clotting, according to the patient's prothrombin ratio. Observation should then be made for signs of bleeding such as haematuria. The leg may be bandaged and bed rest may be ordered, depending on the surgeon's wishes. Oral anticoagulant therapy may also be continued when intravenous therapy has been completed, although there will be an overlap between the discontinuation of heparin and the commencement of oral therapy. Warfarin, for example, will not be active immediately.

Pulmonary embolism may further complicate venous thrombosis; any symptoms of chest pain or signs of breathlessness, sweating, pallor, raised pulse rate or lowered blood pressure should be reported immediately. Medical assistance should be summoned and oxygen administered.

Hygiene

This important facet of care should meet the needs of any individual confined to bed; physical activity may be reduced, but the patient often becomes warm and sweaty and appreciates a cooling wash. It is important to take into consideration the patient's normal hygiene routines and defer to these where possible; any religious observances should also be respected. This is particularly important when bathing becomes possible.

Oral hygiene. Teeth should be cleaned whenever possible with a toothbrush and frequent antiseptic mouth washes should be offered. Dentures may be soaked in proprietary cleaning solutions. If the patient is accustomed to dental flossing, this should be encouraged; if the patient is not accustomed to flossing for the removal of plaque and consequent prevention of dental decay the method should be taught, if possible.

WOUNDS

A wound is a break in the continuity of the skin.

A surgical wound is defined as *clean* if at the time of operation

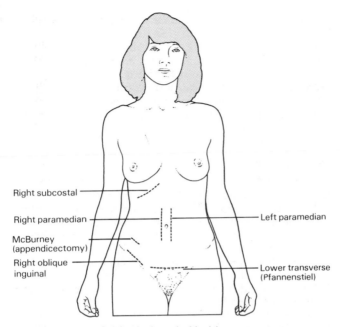

Figure 4. Types of abdominal surgical incision.

there was no inflammation or infection present and no spillage of the contents of a viscus (that is, the viscus had not perforated). A surgical incision (Figure 4) will normally heal by first intention, whereby the edges of the wound are brought into apposition by some form of suturing (primary healing); fibroblastic activity in consequent clot formation results in the laying down of collagen fibres, which in about five days from the initial incision will form early scar tissue.

A wound may be *contaminated*: it may be inflamed and spillage may have occurred, but healing will still be by first intention, with primary suturing, if there is adequate drainage, if the infection can be overcome and if the wound edges can be brought together without loss of tissue.

A *dirty* wound is one in which pus has been encountered or a viscus, for example the appendix, has been found to be perforated.

A wound will heal by *granulation* (epithelialization taking place from its base) if there is gross tissue deficit, for example if a wound has been laid open surgically and the edges either cannot be or are not intended to be, brought into apposition. This type of wound requires skilled attention in order to prevent premature closure at the skin surface, before tissue has grown up from its base. If this happens there may be sinus formation and the prospect of a further surgical incision (this care will be described separately).

Wound drainage

A wound site may require drainage if:
1 Serous fluid is allowed to collect, or a haematoma forms. A focus will be provided for the multiplication of micro-organisms, resulting in infection and tissue breakdown; tissues will not heal when there is an unresolvable collection of fluid.
2 Pus is already present, or the site was found to be contaminated at operation.
3 Bleeding was difficult to control at operation or the area is particularly vascular.

Drainage methods

Closed drainage. A vacuum drainage system may be employed, in which the plastic tubing inserted at the site (and usually sutured in place) is attached to a vacuum bottle or a plastic concertina-type container (Figure 5). There is usually some indication when the vacuum is no longer present and the equipment either needs re-vacuuming or replacing in order to maintain effective suction. Serous fluids are adequately drained in this manner.

Open drainage. Corrugated rubber tubing of various widths may be inserted; this type of drainage tubing may be brought nearer to the skin surface—that is 'shortened'—as the days progress. The reaction of the tubing against the skin surface usually means that a track is formed, through which, after removal of the tubing, drainage will continue if serous fluid or pus are still being produced. The pressure of the tubing on the site can cause tissue necrosis and inhibit healing. Corrugated drainage tubes

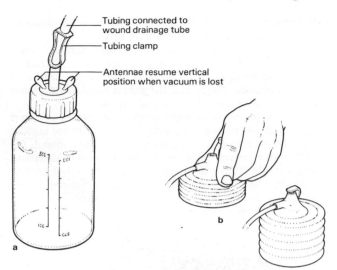

Tubing connected to
wound drainage tube

Tubing clamp

Antennae resume vertical
position when vacuum is lost

b

a

Figure 5. (a) 'Redivac' vacuum bottle closed drainage system. (b)
Lightweight plastic concertina bottle closed drainage system, showing
(bottom) container when vacuum is no longer present. To re-vacuum
empty contents, expel air (top) and close container.

are frequently used in dirty wounds, for example after drainage
of an abscess mass; a stoma bag can be applied to the skin over
the tube or a dressing applied, depending on the amount of
drainage and the condition of the surrounding skin.

Portex or rubber tubing may be inserted for drainage purposes and may either be connected to a drainage bag or simply
allowed to drain its contents into a dressing.

Underwater-seal drainage. This is described on p. 85.

Principles of care
- A vacuum drainage system is only effective if a vacuum is
  always present.
- Tubing should never be clamped off unless there are specific
  instructions to this effect.
- The insertion site must be clean, dry and protected. Drainage
  tubes are frequently inserted through a stab wound, separate

from the main incision, the aim being to prevent contamination of the main incision by drainage tubes.

● Drainage should be observed and charted where and when appropriate, and reported if it is excessive or its characteristics have changed, for example if bile appears instead of sero-sanguineous fluid from the gallbladder bed, or gastric contents appear from the duodenal stump.

● An aseptic technique is required when a corrugated drain is shortened. The tubing will usually have been sutured in place initially; to shorten the tube the suture will be removed, the tubing withdrawn the distance by which it is to be shortened and a sterile safety pin inserted above skin level to prevent the tubing slipping back (Figure 6). A gauze dressing should be placed around the entry site: a keyhole dressing will be comfortable and effective.

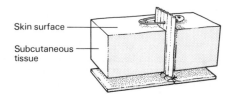

Skin surface
Subcutaneous tissue

Figure 6. Corrugated drainage tube in situ (diagrammatic). When the tube is to be shortened the requisite length is raised above skin level, a sterile pin is re-inserted and excess tubing is cut off.

● Drainage tubes should be removed as directed, generally when drainage is minimal (this is an aseptic procedure). After removal the site should be protected for the first 24 hours and observed for undue drainage thereafter.

Closure of wounds

Cut edges need to be brought into apposition and may be held there by mechanical means—in other words, sutured. The materials used for this purpose will be either absorbable or non-absorbable. Absorbable sutures are made of catgut (sheep's submucosal layer), either plain or chromic (treated with chrome salts to increase its resistance to the effect of enzyme activity and delay its absorption). Non-absorbable sutures include cotton, silk, nylon and wire; they may be mono-filamented or braided.

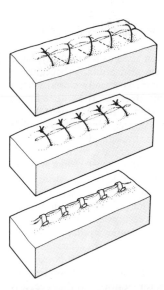

Figure 7. Wound closure: (top) continuous suture, (middle) interrupted sutures, (bottom) clips.

Wounds may be closed by the following types of suture (Figure 7):

1 Continuous suture.
2 Interrupted suture.
3 Subcuticular suture; these are frequently used to close a Pfannenstiel incision (Figure 4) with excellent cosmetic effect.
4 Purse-string suture; this is used to secure, and inserted around, a thoracic drainage tube to be tied off simultaneously with the tube's withdrawal (see Figure 27, p. 90).
5 Stainless steel clips; these are frequently used to close neck incisions, for example after carotid endarterectomy or thyroidectomy; effective closure can be obtained and early removal is possible. Usually alternate clips are removed within 24 hours of the operation and the remainder removed within 48 hours. A special pair of clip-removing forceps is necessary for this procedure (Figure 8).

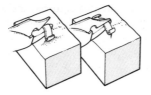

Figure 8. Removal of clips.

Wounds are closed after an operation such as laparotomy, layer by layer—peritoneum, muscle layers and fascia, subcutaneous tissue and skin layer. The peritoneum is usually closed with a continuous catgut suture. If unusual stress on the suture line is anticipated postoperatively, for instance if the patient has a chronic respiratory condition or is obese, deep tension nylon sutures will be inserted at this point, through all the remaining layers, for tying off when all other layers have been separately sutured (rather like the final securing of a parcel). Muscle layers and fascia are closed with either absorbable or non-absorbable suture material, the subcutaneous layer is closed and the skin edges are brought together with nylon. Either continuous or interrupted suturing may be used. Deep tension sutures are tied off after threading through rubber or plastic capillary tubing or over plastic foam pads; the latter protect the skin and the primary suture line from undue pressure caused by postoperative inflammatory oedema and from the possibility of subsequent necrosis. In some areas, for example on the face, it is desirable that, where possible, wound edges are approximated without suturing by strategically placed adherent sterile paper strips (Steri-strips). These are simple to apply, effective for their purpose, reduce skin trauma and the risk of wound infection and produce a good cosmetic effect. The reduction in anxiety and discomfort for the patient, both on application and on removal, will be obvious.

Removal of sutures

In principle, sutures inserted into areas which are not subjected to physical stress and have a good blood supply are removed early—about three days after operation. Abdominal sutures are removed seven to ten days after operation. Lower limb sutures are removed ten days after operation.

However, these are arbitrary periods and the time for the removal of sutures is to a large extent determined by:

1 The circumstances leading to their insertion.
2 The healing characteristics of the individual.
3 The desires of the surgeon: for example, some surgeons will require that, after cardiac surgery, thoracic and lower limb sutures are removed on the same day—about the seventh after the operation.

When sutures are removed:

- An aseptic technique should be used.
- Instruments should be sterile.
- Scissors should be sharp with suitably pointed ends; a stitch cutter may be preferred.
- No suture material above the skin should be allowed to enter or be pulled through the subcutaneous layer after the stitch has been cut.
- A smooth cutting action should be employed.
- The suture should be raised with forceps, thus applying traction on the suture against the skin surface (Figure 9).
- The cutting instrument should be inserted under the suture, flat against the skin surface.
- The suture should be withdrawn towards the incision line.

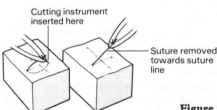

Cutting instrument inserted here

Suture removed towards suture line

Figure 9. Removal of sutures.

Conditions for wound healing

Identification of needs
Physical needs are centred on the patient's:
- Nutritional status
- Circulatory status
- Defence mechanisms and general physical condition

Psychological needs are related to:
- Knowledge of his condition and the reasons for the nursing activities

Related nursing activities

Nutritional status. There have been considerable advances in hospital meal services and there is now a wide choice of menus available and minimal delay between preparation of the food and its presentation at the bedside; however, this sometimes means that the nurse is not aware of the patient's choices and may also not be present when the meal is offered or the tray is eventually removed. It must be the nurse's responsibility to ensure that the patient has foods which will promote wound healing.

1   They must be rich in protein: positive nitrogen balance is essential for tissue repair.

2   They must contain vitamins A and C, for collagen synthesis.

3   They must contain minerals, particularly zinc; these are needed for enzyme activity.

If the patient understands the reasons for essential foods, he is more likely to cooperate in a proper choice. Every effort should be made to suggest suitable alternatives if certain foods are declined for religious or ethnic reasons or simply by personal idiosyncrasy. It is often difficult for patients to drink large amounts of plain water, but other forms of fluid can usually be given such as tea, coffee or other hot beverages, unless these are restricted (for example, on potassium-restricted diets). It is the duty of the nurse to have knowledge of foods forbidden to various ethnic groups, thus avoiding unwittingly giving offence and causing embarrassment.

It is often the case that patients are protein-depleted if food has been restricted preoperatively, and this must be taken into account postoperatively. It may be necessary to restore this and any other deficiency parenterally (see p. 15).

Defence mechanisms and general physical condition. Knowledge of the patient's general condition is essential, as factors other than the immediate surgical problem may delay or complicate healing. For example:

a   If the patient has been receiving steroid therapy he may be slow to heal and the inflammatory response may be masked.

b   If there is a history of diabetes mellitus it may complicate the healing process; this is especially so in patients who undergo surgery to alleviate peripheral vascular disease.

c Obesity is a complicating factor; subcutaneous tissue, containing many fat cells, is difficult to suture.

d Those advanced in years are slow to heal; physical rebound is less certain.

Blood supply. Although ensuring a sufficiency of blood supply to the wound is the province of the surgeon, the nurse is able to promote circulation by some elementary activities:

- Any specific instructions regarding positioning (written in the post-operation notes) must be observed: a limb, for example, may be elevated to reduce the possibility of oedema formation and to assist venous return.
- Undue pressure on the wound from the weight of bedclothes must be relieved with the aid of sheepskins and bed cradles.
- Protection and padding must be provided against hard objects.
- A free, cool circulation of air should be ensured around the wound. A bed cradle may be used for this purpose; it will also relieve unnecessary weight.
- Movement should be encouraged, where appropriate, and any specific exercises explained by the physiotherapist.
- After amputation, special consideration must be given to the circulation in the remaining limb.

A wound will often improve visibly if a low haemoglobin level is rectified by a blood transfusion.

Hygiene. The general hygienic requirements of anyone who has to spend a period in bed must be met. In hospitals these requirements are accentuated as hospital beds are invariably protected by much plastic covering, which keeps heat in and causes excessive sweating. Moreover, non-pathogens normally found on the skin may become pathogenic in the patient at risk—the surgical patient, whose skin surface is no longer intact. A blanket bath, efficiently performed, is therapeutic for this reason alone, but it also allows time for patient contact which may not otherwise be available.

Rest and sleep. These aids are essential to cell regeneration. Both can be promoted if the patient is relatively free from immediately obvious, anxiety-raising situations. Every effort must be made to provide explanations for all procedures relating to the management of a wound, and sufficient time and opportunity must be allowed for questions to be asked and answered.

Prevention of wound infection

Identification of needs
- A safe ward environment
- Care directly related to the surgical incision

A safe ward environment

Related nursing activities
In most hospitals, the responsibility for cleaning no longer rests with the nursing staff but rests with persons trained to supervise ancillary staff in the maintenance of acceptable standards. Although relieved of this responsibility, nurses must be aware of those factors which may expose the patient to the risks inherent in a wound infection. Some general factors, if rigidly observed, lessen the risk of infection on the surgical ward.
- Furniture and equipment should not be shared.
- Bowls, tooth mugs and so on should be disposable or be autoclaved; if this type of equipment is not available, items must be properly washed, thoroughly dried and separately stacked.
- Bed linen should be changed frequently and disposed of according to hospital policy. The linen bin must be brought to the bedside. Soiled linen should not be carried against the uniform.
- Bed pans and commodes need to be clean and dry (this is an aesthetic consideration as well as an infection hazard).
- Sticky surfaces (caused by spilt fruit juices, for example) must be avoided.
- Flower vases should be emptied at a sink away from the clinical area.
- Sitting on a patient's bed is not a good nursing practice; effective communication is possible sitting at the bedside. Communication is concerned with content, eye contact and many other non-verbal activities. Sitting on the bed can be interpreted as an invasion of the patient's territory and his privacy. Furthermore, in the context of the prevention of infection, bacteria are present in desquamated cells in the bedclothes and may be transmitted in this manner.

- Isolation policies should be observed; all ward personnel should be conversant with the procedures practised in their institution.

The nurse has responsibilities to:

- The patient. Wound infection will delay healing, increase discomfort, and may result in failure of the surgical procedure (for example, a skin graft may not take) or even a fatal outcome. It will delay discharge home and possibly result in financial hardship (such as loss of earnings) and considerable domestic upset.
- Herself. A sound knowledge of (a) the sources of possible infection, (b) the mode of transmission of organisms and (c) the means of prevention are essential. She must recognize herself as a potential source of cross-infection and attend conscientiously to her personal hygiene and health.

    The nurse has a role as a health educator, and should take every opportunity available to promote good hygienic practices in regard to patients, their relatives and other members of the caring team.
- The institution. An unnecessarily prolonged hospital stay for one patient can reduce another's opportunities for treatment and dilute available financial resources.

    As a local institution, a hospital's reputation rests on its service to its community; this is reflected in the confidence placed in it by that community. This confidence is fragile, easily undermined by adverse reports of standards of care.

In relation to the control of infection, the 'control of infection nurse' has a firmly established role to play as an active and invaluable member of the caring team. She is able to identify patients at risk, can offer specialist advice, supported by research findings, and liaises with laboratory personnel.

Nursing care of the patient with a surgical incision

Identification of needs

Inflammation is a local reaction by the body tissues in response to injury: a surgical incision demonstrates this immediate response. Inflammation is characterized by an increase in the volume of blood flowing to the affected area but a decrease in the rate of flow *through* it, by capillary permeability and hence by accumulation of fluid in the extracellular spaces. The area consequently feels hot, looks red, appears swollen and is painful; depending on the site affected, function may be impaired. The patient will have a raised temperature and will feel unwell; the white cell count will also be raised (normal: $4-11 \times 10^9$ per litre).The inflammation will, however, resolve and healing will take place, providing pathogenic organisms are prevented from invading the wound.

If pathogens have gained access to the wound, or if a focus for the inflammatory response is inadvertently permitted to remain—for example, suture material is left in an incision—infection is said to be present, and this can be confirmed by laboratory culture of the exudate present at the site. The causative organism can be identified and its sensitivity to a range of antimicrobial drugs ascertained. Subsequent drug treatment will depend on the result of this investigation.

The patient may develop a septicaemia, when organisms are present in the blood; this is a serious condition in which the temperature is elevated, as is the white cell count. The patient may also experience the distressing symptoms of a rigor, which is the attempt by temperature-regulating mechanisms to adjust the general body temperature to that of a greatly raised core temperature; this is characterized by uncontrollable episodes of shivering.

Nursing activities related to the prevention of wound infection
- The patient should be allowed some responsibility for his own well-being, related to the incision. This requires that he be instructed on the need for cleanliness and given an explanation of how organisms which may not be harmful in one area of his body may become so in another, if elementary hygiene rules are not followed. His desire to inspect a wound is a natural one but should be resisted; this will be easier to accept if the reasons are explained.
- He must be encouraged to report any discomfort at the site and any sudden or excessive oozing which may make a protective dressing wet and allow access for bacteria.
- Before any dressing is undertaken, the patient must be prepared. It may be the first occasion on which what appears to the patient as an unsightly wound is exposed; fears and anxieties, if expressed, can be alleviated by quiet reassurances during the procedure. Analgesia should be offered

prior to any uncomfortable procedure. An individual's height-ened awareness of smells should be acknowledged, even though undue body odour may not be apparent to the nurse.
- Hand washing is the principal precaution to be taken against wound cross-infection; bactericidal solutions such as chlor-hexidine are suitable for this purpose, but hand washing will not be effective unless meticulous attention is also paid to hand drying.

Management of the wound
- The principles of asepsis, using a non-touch technique, should be employed throughout.
- The wound should be carefully assessed and all equipment and solutions collected together before the wound is exposed; minimal time should be permitted between exposure and completion of the procedure.
- Activity at the bed area should be minimal and dressings are often more safely carried out in an area specifically set aside for this purpose.
- Surgical incisions should be kept dry. If cleaning is con-sidered necessary and an aqueous solution has been used, the suture line must be carefully dried before a dressing is applied.
- Dressings should be adequate for protection, where necessary, and comfort.
- Strapping should be applied, taking into consideration the shape of the patient, the position of the wound and the amount of movement possible. Movement should not be restricted, unless this is the object of the strapping or bandag-ing. The patient's comments regarding comfort and any known allergic response to specific types of adhesive plasters should be noted and responded to accordingly.
- Many surgical incisions are left exposed and sprayed with a plastic dressing. It is possible to take a shower earlier with this type of dressing, if the patient wishes and his condition permits it.
- If a wound becomes infected:
  a Early recognition is important: the wound may ooze and pus may be present.
  b Some sutures may be removed to facilitate drainage if the wound breaks down.
  c Dead tissue must be removed before healing is possible.

Eusol is often used for this desloughing but precautions must be taken to prevent its application to surrounding healthy tissue, where it will continue its activity.

- Some surgeons require their patients to immerse an infected wound in a bath; if this is to be done it is the nurse's responsibility to ensure that the bath is thoroughly cleaned each time it is used and some thought should be given as to the nature of the wound infection and its mode of transmission.
- Hydrogen peroxide may be used to irrigate a wound.
- If healing is to proceed by granulation a wound may be lightly packed with sterile ribbon gauze, to prevent early closure before healing has taken place from the base of the wound. The ribbon gauze, if kept moist, will accelerate epithelialization. A note should be made on the care plan of the amount of gauze used for the dressing, to prevent a portion being overlooked and not removed when the dressing is next renewed.
- A clear description of the appearance of the wound should be written, either in a Kardex or in a continuing plan of care. The progress of the wound and the effectiveness of treatment can be evaluated and further care planned accordingly.

Debridement. Some wounds may need to be radically treated by removal of necrotic tissue; this is usually carried out under anaesthetic.

STERILIZATION

Many items of ward equipment are sterilized before use; the term means the destruction of all living organisms, and this can be achieved in a number of different ways.

Autoclaving. Items to be autoclaved are loosely wrapped in paper and sealed with a heat-sensitive tape. Air is pumped from the autoclave machine, steam is introduced under pressure and air and steam are removed mechanically at the end of the cycle. The sterilizing temperature is usually about 136°C and the cycle may vary in time from a few minutes to about 30 minutes, depending on the size of the machine. Many cotton dressing materials and items such as rubber suction catheters and metal and plastic forceps may be autoclaved, but assembled plastic syringes are not effectively sterilized by this method, because steam must reach every surface.

Ethylene oxide. This is used to sterilize large pieces of equipment and those which may be damaged by heat. Contaminated rooms can be sterilized in this way: the gas is released into the atmosphere.

Infra-red heating. Infra-red rays give no visible light but produce heat. A temperature of 180°C can be attained and is held for about ten minutes. Glass syringes and instruments are sometimes sterilized in this manner.

Ionizing radiation. Gamma radiation is used commercially and most pre-packed articles, including suture materials, and rubber and plastic equipment, are sterilized in this way.

Related nursing activities
● Any autoclaved pack intended for a sterile procedure must be rejected if the pack is damaged in any way—if it is not intact or is wet. The tape used to seal the pack will change colour when it has been autoclaved; this must be checked.
● Packs are sealed in such a way that the contents can be removed from the bags in which they are contained without being contaminated. The method must be understood and complied with on every occasion.

DISINFECTANTS

Disinfectants are chemical substances used for the destruction of pathogenic organisms. Most hospitals and similar institutions have specific policies governing their use which have been evolved through consultation with laboratory staff and control-of-infection staff.

The following are examples of commonly used disinfectants:

Ethanol. Surfaces used for aseptic or clean procedures may be washed with soap and water to remove organic matter, and subsequently sprayed with methylated spirit at a concentration of 70%; ethanol (ethyl alcohol) wipes are also available for this purpose. The surface should be allowed to dry by evaporation before it is used.

Chlorhexidine. Solutions of chlorhexidine are bacteriostatic and bactericidal against a wide range of organisms and can be used for skin and wound cleaning. They may also be added to nasal creams for use in preoperative preparations, preventing nasal carriage of staphylococci.

Chlorine-releasing solutions. Milton (sodium hypochlorite) may be used to disinfect equipment (especially infant feeding equipment). Eusol is frequently used to deslough necrotic areas, but precautions must be taken to prevent its application onto surrounding healthy tissue.

Oxidizing agents. Hydrogen peroxide may be used to irrigate wounds; oxygen is released at the site and its bubbling action removes wound debris and pus.

Phenolic disinfectants. These, appropriately diluted, are employed for cleaning drains, sinks and so on.

Related nursing activities
- Most careful attention must be paid to the instructions for use of any solutions.
- Disinfectants are only effective if correctly diluted in the appropriate solution and at the correct temperature.
- Articles will only be disinfected if they are totally immersed for the correct time and the solutions are changed as directed.
- The utmost care must be taken in handling any solutions, some of which may be corrosive or will burn. Gloves should be used when handling phenolic disinfectants.
- All containers should be stored in locked cupboards and out of the reach of children.

NURSING THE PATIENT IN ISOLATION

It is sometimes necessary to nurse patients in isolation, or at least to take precautions not normally required, when assisting the patient or handling soiled objects or body fluids. The following are some of the reasons for this type of procedure.

Some organisms become resistant to a range of antimicrobial drugs normally used in hospitals and can cause serious problems if permitted to spread to other patients (cross-infection).

Some organisms are capable of producing toxins and may go on to cause septicaemia or renal or cardiac complications if transmitted to patients at risk, for example those whose normal defence mechanisms are already being challenged; such an organism is group A haemolytic *Streptococcus*.

Some patients are HBsAg positive: that is, they carry the hepatitis B virus in their body fluids.

Patients may need to be protected from other patients and ward staff when being treated with certain drugs. Some therapeutic agents—cytotoxic drugs—will reduce the patient's white cell count and consequently make him more vulnerable to infection. Hospital policy varies regarding which patients are to be isolated, and the methods to be employed, but written guidelines are usually available and advice can always be obtained from a control-of-infection nurse.

Identification of needs
- Physical protection of all those at risk
- Psychological support for the isolated patient and his relatives

Related nursing activities
- Knowledge of mode of transmission of organisms. It is essential to know whether the infection for which the patient has been isolated:

  a   is spread by direct contact—for instance, by bed linen in contact with a wound;

  b   is airborne—for example, tubercle bacillus;

  c   is present in body fluids—for example hepatitis B virus in blood.

  The mode of transmission will determine the policy to be followed and whether gowns, masks and/or gloves will be worn.
- Equipment. All equipment must be thoughtfully assembled in the patient's room.

- There should be some indication that isolation precautions are needed on entering the room.
- Hand washing. This is an essential element in care.
- Disposal of potentially contaminated equipment and bed linen. Double-bagging procedures are frequently adopted; some items may need to be labelled before disposal.
- Specimens for investigation purposes. These must be clearly labelled and correctly transported; the health of many other individuals outside the immediate ward area may be in jeopardy if labelling is inadequate.
- Items to be disinfected. Instructions for dilution of disinfecting agents must be carefully followed. Many items such as plates, cups and other utensils are now disposable; this will reduce the need to soak articles.
- Protection of ancillary staff. Many hospitals have instituted short training courses for cleaning staff, who are involved indirectly in patient care. There is a responsibility on nursing staff to protect the ancillary staff from risk and to deal effectively with any contingency that may arise as a result of insufficient knowledge of aspects of care. Room cleaning is as essential for the patient's well-being as many other aspects of care.
- Psychological support. Patients who are nursed in isolation are often deprived of the normal social interaction that a ward environment offers. They may already be feeling ill and become withdrawn and morose. Conversation may only be possible through masks, and physical contact is often through plastic aprons, gloves and so on. Eating and drinking, normally an enjoyable social occasion, is a solitary non-stimulating affair, with food on a plastic plate, eaten with a plastic knife and fork. Every opportunity to decrease sensory deprivation must be taken and mental diversions such as a radio, paperback books and newspapers must be provided. A few minutes spent in conversation, explaining procedures and answering questions, or simply talking about the weather, can be invaluable. The forgotten cup of tea is unforgivable.
- Isolation in the open ward. There may be no suitable room available for isolation nursing, but it is possible to carry out stringent, safe, precautionary nursing in an open ward area, with the support and advice of the control-of-infection nurse, whose expertise should always be sought.

- Strict isolation. There are some rare diseases with a high mortality rate (for example, Lassa fever) which require strict isolation techniques, away from a general hospital. Specific establishments are available for this purpose and special precautions are taken if such a disease is suspected.

Relatives and friends

Identification of needs
- It is important that those concerned with the patient's future well-being are involved in all stages of care, both physical and psychological. Insight into the patient's needs may only be achieved by those intimately involved in his normal activities of daily living.

Related nursing activities
- Information regarding daily progress (and setbacks) must be readily available. Telephone conversations should be informative, relating details of progress, which even if they may appear minimal, have relevance and express human concern.
- The stress and anxieties experienced by those intimately concerned with the patient must be recognized. Behaviour which may appear aggressive or inconsiderate must be met with courtesy and understanding at all times.

PREPARATION FOR DISCHARGE

The time spent in a hospital after undergoing comparatively major surgical procedures may be as little as ten days, whilst some patients may even be discharged on the same day as they undergo surgery. This is possible providing the patient's postoperative recovery is considered satisfactory and the domestic conditions to which he will return are adequate for his postoperative needs.

Some principles must be observed when discharge is imminent; the nurse responsible for discharging the patient has certain obligations. She is responsible to:

1 The patient and his relatives: for ensuring that reasonable provision is made and foreseeable difficulties are anticipated.

2 The institution and her colleagues: for ensuring that the

institution is not brought into disrepute by inadequate preparation for discharge.

3 Society: for ensuring that health care resources are effectively used. Society provides for health care for all in time of need and the need may continue for some time after the patient has been discharged.

Discharge may be to one of many places, including:

a The patient's own home
b A convalescent home
c A new home with relatives
d Residential accommodation
e Another ward which cares for the elderly when independence is no longer possible.

Support may consequently be forthcoming from: relatives, the social services, and the primary health care team. On the other hand, total independence may have been achieved and needs on discharge may be minimal.

Identification of needs
Sufficient time must be allowed for:

- Physical preparation—for example, making transport arrangements, obtaining equipment or apparatus.
- Psychological preparation—such as adjustment to changed body image or re-entry into society after many months in a relatively sheltered and ordered environment.
- Social preparation.

Related nursing activities
Patient education should aim to promote a full recovery where possible or, where this is not realistic, to enhance the quality of life which remains. There are many nurse specialists who are able to offer advice and sometimes support the patient when he returns home; these include:

a the nurse nutritionist
b the control of infection nurse
c the stoma therapist
d nurses who are skilled in counselling
e nurses whose expertise is devoted to the terminally ill

Advice should be offered regarding:

1 Diet. Some items may be restricted or undesirable and

sound reasons should be given for such restrictions, reinforced where possible by literature and the services of a dietician.

2 Rest/exercise/work. Advice should be explicit, couched in terms the patient will understand; rest will have a different meaning for people pursuing different occupations.

3 Medication. Any drugs to be taken away should be clearly labelled by the pharmacy department and verbal instructions reinforced by written instructions if necessary. If the drugs are to be administered or supervised by a third party, that person should be present when the instructions are given.

- The date and time of follow-up appointments should be discussed with the patient before the appointment is made and the details should be clearly written down. Appointments early in the day may be difficult for elderly people to keep and another consideration affecting the timing of the appointment must be the availability of transport for the patient or his relatives.
- Facilities should be available for contact to be maintained between the patient and the ward, thus promoting a feeling of security and continuing support.
- The patient's general practitioner must always be informed of the patient's discharge, of any treatment which has been undertaken and the drugs which have been prescribed (this is usually the responsibility of the surgical team).
- Psychological adjustment. The process of assisting the patient towards acceptance and adjustment should begin before surgery is undertaken, but this ideal may not always be possible. As the time for return to society draws near, after surgery which has altered body image, such as amputation or formation of a colostomy, behaviour changes may indicate unspoken anxieties and apprehension. The nurse must be sensitive to this situation and help to promote a positive attitude at this testing time. Skilled counsellors are available to assist in this nursing objective.

Support available in the community

The community nurse. The community nurse will visit the patient, in his home if necessary, carrying out dressing procedures, administering injections and so on. The initial treatment may be given according to the advice received from the ward on which the patient was treated, but afterwards the patient's treatment will be a matter to be decided between the community nurse, the general practitioner and the patient. The patient should be given sufficient dressings for the community nurse to carry out an initial dressing before she makes her own assessment of need.

The social services. Certain services are available to all members of the community in need:

1 Meals on Wheels provides an adequate nourishing hot meal; this is sometimes cooked and distributed by local voluntary groups, but the service is financed through the Social Services Department of the local authority.

2 A home help service undertakes light household chores, shopping, and other tasks.

3 Various household fitments, such as doorways, toilet seat height and taps, may be adapted and some items ordered to promote mobility.

4 Financial provision is also available for special dietary needs and surgical equipment.

5 Laundry and disposal services are provided by some councils.

6 Arrangements can be made with many chemist's shops for the regular supply of special equipment, such as that for the management of a colostomy or ileostomy.

The resources available may be dependent on the patient's own financial status; however, advice is available at health centres and at local authority offices.

Further reading

Abdellah, F.G., Beland, I.L., Martin, A. & Matheney, R.V. (1960) *Patient-centred Approaches to Nursing* New York: Macmillan.

Bower, F.L. & Bevis, E.O. (1979) *Fundamentals of Nursing Practice* St Louis: Mosby.

Henderson, V. (1966) *The Nature of Nursing: A Definition and its Implications for Practice, Research and Education* New York: Macmillan.

Kratz, C.R. (Ed.) (1979) *The Nursing Process* London: Baillière Tindall.

Orem, D.E. (1980) *Nursing—Concept and Practice* New York: McGraw-Hill.

Riehl, J. & Roy, C. (1974) *Conceptual models for nursing practice* New York: Appleton-Century-Crofts.

Roper, N., Logan, W.W. & Tierney, A. (1980) *The Elements of Nursing* Edinburgh: Churchill Livingstone.

Pharmacology
Turner, P. & Richens, A. (1982) *Clinical Pharmacology,* 4th edition. Edinburgh: Churchill Livingstone.

Anaesthesia
Wachstein, J. & Smith, J.A.H. (1981) *Anaesthesia and Recovery Room Techniques,* 3rd edition (Nurses' Aids Series—Special Interest Text). London: Baillière Tindall.

Pain
Hayward, J. (1975) *Information—A Prescription against Pain* London: Royal College of Nursing.
McCaffrey, M. (1972) *Nursing Management of the Patient With Pain* Philadelphia: Lippincott.
Coping with Pain (part 1) (1979) *Nursing* (April).

Intravenous therapy
British Journal of Parenteral Therapy
Department of Health and Social Security (1976) *Addition of Drugs to Intravenous Infusion Fluids* DHSS Circular HC(76)9 (March 1976).
Grant, G. & Todd, E. (1982) *Enteral and Parenteral Nutrition* Oxford: Blackwell Scientific.
Willats, S.M. (1982) *Lecture Notes on Fluid and Electrolyte Balance* Oxford: Blackwell Scientific.

Wounds
Westaby, S. (Ed.) (1982) Wound Care Series. *Nursing Times.*

Nursing in isolation
Winner, H.I. (1978) *Microbiology in Patient Care,* 2nd edition. London: Hodder & Stoughton.

Discharge
Wilson-Barnett, J. (Ed.) (1983) *Patient Teaching* Edinburgh: Churchill Livingstone.

2
Breast Surgery

The breasts are situated on either side of the sternum, over the 2nd to 6th ribs. They lie in superficial fascia, separated from the deep fascia overlying the pectoralis major muscle by loose connective tissue, which allows for some movement of the breast over it. They are composed of glandular, fibrous and fatty tissue and are stabilized by ligaments. Each breast is divided into lobes, which are separated by fibrous tissue (Figure 10).

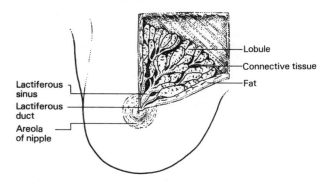

Figure 10. The breast: structure.

The blood supply is from the internal and external mammary arteries, while the venous return is via the internal mammary veins and the axillary veins. Three-quarters of the lymphatic drainage is into the axillary nodes and one-quarter is into the para-sternal nodes.

Hormonal changes take place in the breasts and premenstrual symptoms—fullness, heaviness and discomfort—are frequently experienced. After the menopause the breast regresses and becomes more fibrous.

Benign conditions

Breast lumps may be benign and less than one in four women who are investigated are found to have breast cancer. The benign lump is discrete and never gives rise to metastases. It may be derived from various tissues of the breast. Thus, a lipoma is derived from fat cells and a fibroadenoma arises from glandular and fibrous tissue. A cyst is a collection of fluid within a capsule, which may be sufficiently tense to form a hard lump.

Breast cancer

Each year 12 000 women in Great Britain die from cancer of the breast and it is the commonest cause of death in females between the ages of 35 and 55. While the ten-year survival rate improved between 1920 and 1950, the rate has not changed significantly since that date. There appears to be increasing public awareness of the life-threatening nature of the disease and there are some recognized predisposing factors, which may help to identify those women at risk:

1   There is a familial tendency.
2   Single women have a high incidence of breast cancer.
3   Late pregnancy is known to increase the risk.
4   There are definite geographical variations, with a high incidence in Western Europe and USA and an extremely low incidence in South East Asia.

Studies have so far failed to show a definite relationship between taking the contraceptive pill and breast cancer.

Malignant breast lumps are usually hard and irregular, painless and fixed to the skin. There may be skin changes. Infiltration of tumour along the fibrous divisions of the breast blocks lymphatic drainage and causes oedema of the overlying skin between the hair follicles and the sweat glands; the appearance is that of orange peel—'peau d'orange'. Axillary nodes may be enlarged.

The Manchester classification of carcinoma of the breast identifies clinical signs which if present may determine treatment and predict a possible outcome:

Stage I   the disease is confined to the breast
Stage II   regional lymph nodes are also involved
Stage III   underlying tissue is involved: this is locally advanced disease

Stage IV   metastases are present

Stages I and II are usually considered operable, but stages III and IV will not respond to surgery. Radiotherapy and adjuvant systemic therapy may be considered where disease has spread via the lymphatic system or the blood.

Investigations

Some of the following procedures may need to be carried out in order to exclude malignancy or to determine the extent of the disease process:

1   Aspiration biopsy: removal of fluid by syringe and needle for cytology.

2   Needle biopsy: insertion of a cutting needle and removal of a core of material for histopathological examination.

Aspiration and needle biopsy are carried out under local anaesthetic.

3   Mammography: a soft tissue X-ray, which can show changes that are not clinically detectable.

4   Thermography. An infra-red scanner is used to measure heat emission from an abnormal vascular pattern. This investigation may show a false positive result.

5   Excision biopsy. This is done under general anaesthetic.

Evidence of metastases may be determined by ultrasonography, skeletal survey and scanning.

Related nursing activities

The female breasts have cultural and sexual significance and the prospect of possible mutilating surgery may be overwhelming for the woman concerned and any partner. The nurse may frequently need to assess her own responses, and her aim must be one of positive emotional and physical support, throughout both investigation and treatment.

● Time must be made for listening and the nurse who is able to detect non-verbal signs of distress is a great asset to a ward.

Surgery

The following procedures may be undertaken:

1   Lumpectomy: removal of the lump only

2   Simple mastectomy: removal of the breast

3   Modified radical mastectomy: removal of the breast plus the axillary nodes

The more radical operation, involving removal of the pectoral muscles together with the breast and the axillary contents is now rarely performed.

The aims of nursing care
- A successful physical outcome implies that the wound heals uneventfully, without fluid collecting under the suture line or oedema formation (which can occur if axillary nodes are dissected).
- Mental tranquillity is an important patient need.

Related nursing activities—preoperative
- Anxiety and stress may be lessened by night sedation and perhaps a drug to reduce tension during the day, if desired (e.g. diazepam 5 mg three times a day).
- Skin preparation may include an axillary shave where necessary.
- Clear information on the postoperative limitations of arm movement is needed. The extent of exercise desired is dependent on the surgeon; some restrict movement immediately postoperatively, whereas others place no restriction on normal activity.

Related nursing activities—postoperative
- A prime nursing responsibility is the prevention of oedema of the arm, which may result from venous and lymphatic stasis if axillary nodes have been dissected. The arm should be comfortably elevated on pillows.
- A pressure dressing will be in situ; this should be observed for undue oozing.
- Any drainage system (for example, the closed vacuum 'Redivac' type may be used), must always be functioning; inadequate drainage may result in early haematoma or serous fluid collection under the suture line.
- Positive psychological support is essential; from the first moments after recovery from the anaesthetic, the patient will invariably want to know the extent of the surgery performed.
- Adequate analgesia should always be available.

Continuing care
- An immaculate personal appearance is often very important and this interest should be encouraged as soon as appropriate.

- Gentle normal arm movements should be encouraged, according to the surgeon's wishes.
- The dressing will normally be removed on about the third day. This may be a traumatic moment and the patient should be properly prepared. A light dressing should be reapplied.
- Drainage tubes will remain until there is minimal drainage, between five and seven days after surgery.
- Sutures are removed on the 10th to 14th day after surgery.
- Support may be available from other patients on the ward; they are often the key to a positive response.
- A lightweight temporary prosthesis should be provided for the period that the scar is tender and vulnerable.
- Cytotoxic drugs may be administered as part of a planned programme of postoperative treatment. The patient may feel very nauseated, may vomit and be anorectic; the effect and side-effects of the drugs must be carefully explained and the symptoms treated (for example, with antiemetics such as metoclopramide 10 mg i.m.). The patient should be offered fluids and small portions of light foods, not too highly flavoured or pungent in smell.

Future health considerations
- Radiotherapy may be given as an outpatient procedure.
- Advice on the more permanent prostheses should be readily available. The Mastectomy Association has members who are trained in counselling and giving advice on prostheses and their suitability.
- Regular follow-up appointments should be made at which the breasts will be examined and the arms checked for lymphoedema.
- 30% of all women who have cancer of the breast also develop depressive illness and may need skilled counselling. Support must also be considered for other members of the family.
- The advent of screening clinics and the increasing dissemination of information relating to early, regular breast examination are positive moves towards recognizing the social significance of this condition.

Further reading

Baum, M. (1981) *Breast Cancer—The Facts* Oxford: Oxford Medical Publications.

3
Plastic Surgery

The aim of plastic operations is the correction of deformity by reconstruction ('plastic' is from the Greek *plastikos,* meaning 'capable of being formed or moulded'), and in recent years the opportunity to perfect these procedures has been immense. The rudimentary repair of congenital facial defects in order to preserve life is not new, but the Second World War presented an opportunity for many innovations and improvements in surgical techniques (as wars are wont to do). Other factors which have facilitated this progress have been the rising incidence of injuries sustained in traffic accidents, the more radical methods used to remove malignant tumours and the ability to sustain life in those who, in earlier times, would not have survived to require plastic surgery (for example, victims of severe burns, with extensive tissue loss).

Plastic procedures now cross the boundaries of general surgery, and those skilled in the art are able to advise in many areas where gross disfigurement and loss of function are no longer acceptable to the patient or the surgeon.

This chapter is concerned mainly with those aspects of plastic surgery involving free skin grafting and refers briefly to flap transfers and special points of nursing care relating to them.

Free skin grafts. An area in which granulation is taking place will generally accept a free skin graft, that is, one which is completely detached from the donor site and applied to a recipient area. These are of two types:

1 *Split skins:* epidermis plus a variable part of the dermis (Figure 11). Possible donor site: lateral aspect of the thigh.
2 *Full thickness:* epidermis and full thickness of dermis. Possible donor site: back of pinna.

Skin flaps. When the recipient area is not sufficiently vascular to support a free skin graft, and the grafted skin, in order to be viable, needs to receive a blood supply from the donor site, a flap may be raised. This is a full thickness of epidermis and dermis,

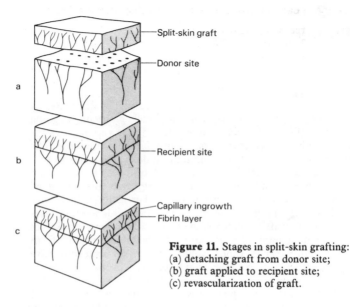

Figure 11. Stages in split-skin grafting:
(a) detaching graft from donor site;
(b) graft applied to recipient site;
(c) revascularization of graft.

plus fat, which remains attached at its proximal end to the donor site while being sutured at its distant end to the recipient area.

This flap may simply be rotated to an adjacent recipient area, for example from the buttock to sacral area to cover a tissue deficit resulting from a pressure sore; this is the *rotation flap*. Alternatively, the graft may be transposed via an intervening area in stages when the distance is impossible to bridge in one procedure, because of problems with the viability of the graft and the physical tolerance of the patient; this is the *pedicle graft*. For example, one end of a flap which is to be taken from the abdominal wall and transferred to the lower limb may be attached to the wrist, from which it is supplied with blood, before being detached from the abdomen; the flap, still attached to the wrist, is then attached to the final recipient site. It is detached from the wrist when viable. The donor site will be closed by primary suturing or a split skin graft.

Nursing care of the patient undergoing skin grafting

The degree to which the graft is successful is described as the 'take'. There are some important points to be borne in mind which are related to nursing care. As a general rule capillary distribution is greater at the upper surface of the dermis (Figure 11), and the thinner the layer of dermis grafted, the more chance there will be of a successful take. In the initial stages the graft is dependent for its nutrition on the fibrinous exudate from the recipient area, but within 48–72 hours, provided the graft is immobile, capillary buds on the surface of the recipient area will grow into the donor skin.

Identification of needs

The aim of nursing care is to preserve the graft, and some essential conditions must exist before surgery is carried out.

- The patient needs to be aware of the conditions necessary for a successful take, the extent of the donor site and of the possibility that the early result may not be immediately cosmetically acceptable.
- The recipient area needs to be in a suitable condition to receive skin, free from infection and from necrotic material, which is likely to be present in chronic venous ulceration which has failed to heal spontaneously.

Related nursing activities—preoperative

- The nurse is able to give the patient information about the donor site; this is often an extensive area and always securely bandaged postoperatively. The tops of the dermal papillae are cut off when the donor skin is removed and quite severe bleeding may occur immediately, but this ceases on the application of a pressure dressing. The area is also very uncomfortable postoperatively, always more so than the recipient area.
- The donor area must be shaved and clean.
- The recipient site may need regular cleaning or a desloughing agent may be used prior to surgery. These substances, for example Eusol, if prescribed, should be used with care, as damage to surrounding skin can easily occur. Ideally the site should be kept moist with normal saline or sterile water immediately prior to surgery.
- The site should be free of infection; *Streptococcus pyogenes,*

for example, is fibrinolytic and its presence is undesirable. A wound swab may be taken and a systemic antimicrobial drug may be prescribed if microorganisms are isolated.

● A major concern is stability of the recipient site postoperatively. If the mechanism of 'take' is described to the patient, possible problems of postoperative mobility may be largely eliminated.

Related nursing activities—postoperative
The aim is to prevent, by skilful care, those occurrences which will cause the graft to be rejected. It is important, therefore, to read the patient's surgical notes carefully for any special instructions which may relate to restriction of movement.

● The recipient area should be protected from undue pressure from bed linen; dressings which usually consist of tulle gras (paraffin gauze dressing) covered by cotton wool applied with uniform pressure and secured by a crêpe bandage, should be inspected regularly.

● Analgesia must be given as often as necessary to relieve the discomfort arising from the donor site.

● The dressing on the recipient area will not be removed for about five days, or according to instruction, when removing the first dressing great care is needed not to remove the graft as well! Sometimes a proflavine (flavine) wool pad is sewn over the graft, providing a uniform pressure dressing and complete stability. If the surgeon has chosen to graft the area and leave it exposed, even more care will be needed to protect it from inadvertent damage, such as rubbing off. It is sometimes helpful to fix a pad round the area to prevent this happening.

Continuing care
● The graft will not take if serosanguineous fluid is allowed to collect under the graft (forming a haematoma); this should be removed and small blisters cut, observing aseptic principles. Any grafted skin which overlaps the raw edges should be trimmed to the size of the grafted area. The area is usually re-dressed with tulle gras cut to size, and carefully bandaged.

● The early recognition of infection is very important and any rise in temperature should be reported.

● Extra donor skin is sometimes saved and can be applied over areas where the initial graft is rejected. Skin may be kept for about 21 days at a temperature of 4°C and is stored, rolled in gauze, in a container of isotonic saline. It is usually placed dermal side uppermost to facilitate application.

- The dressing on the donor site remains in situ for 10 to 14 days; it tends to stick to the area and become somewhat hardened with old blood and exudate. The patient is often sensitive to its distinctive smell and the situation may be helped by frequent changes of bed linen and circulating fresh air.

- The dressing is most easily removed in a bath and this is usually very welcome to the patient, although when water touches the site initially it can be very uncomfortable. An oral analgesic prior to the bath will help overcome this. The site should be clean and pink when the dressing is removed and another light dressing may be needed to protect it from bed clothes, but ideally it should be exposed if possible. The area will heal quickly without scarring; a light massage with arachis oil can relieve the problem of dryness and tightness around the area.

- Once the donor dressing has been removed, the patient should be encouraged to be as active as his general condition allows.

Skin flaps

Distal flaps—those which involve moving tissue at a distance from the primary defect—may take many weeks of bed rest to complete.

Related nursing activities

- Immobility can be a real problem, psychologically as well as physically; the patient will be anxious and in need of constant reassurance that he is positioned correctly.

- Comfort may be difficult to achieve, especially if limbs are splinted, but is always possible with imagination and judicious use of pillows, sheepskins, foam pads and so on.

- Psychological distress may be helped with a small regular dose of a minor tranquillizer if the patient so desires.

- Constant observation should be kept for early signs of ischaemic changes, discolouration or oedema; the flap should never be under undue tension or be kinked and any suction should always be functioning adequately.

Further reading

Harvey Kemble, J.V. & Lamb, B.E. (1984) *Plastic Surgical and Burns Nursing* (Current Nursing Practice Series). London: Baillière Tindall.

McGregor, I.A. (1960) *Fundamental Techniques of Plastic Surgery*. Edinburgh: Churchill Livingstone.

4
Vascular Surgery

ARTERIAL SURGERY

Arterial by-pass surgery of the lower limb

Generalized atherosclerotic changes resulting in narrowing of the lumen of the arteries (especially at bifurcations of vessels) and consequent reduction in blood flow to the lower limb (Figures 12 and 13) have been shown to be closely associated with cigarette smoking. Of the patients who complain of pain in the legs, which is indicative of the disease, 95% are smokers. Advances in technology and surgical techniques have resulted in by-pass operations that are significantly more successful, particularly those involving the larger arteries. It is often possible to by-pass iliac or femoral vessels if there is severe obstruction to arterial flow, and to provide an adequate circulation to the lower limb. This by-pass may lessen the possibility of eventual amputation resulting from irreversible ischaemic changes (Figures 14, 15 and 16).

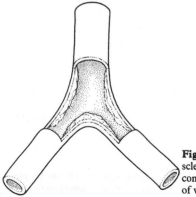

Figure 12. Generalized atherosclerotic changes, which are commonly found at bifurcations of vessels.

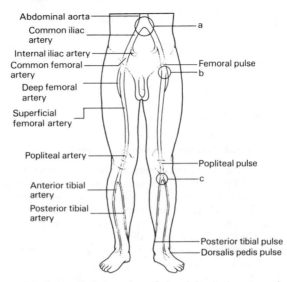

Figure 13. Lower-limb branches of the abdominal aorta and pulse points. (a), (b) and (c): common sites of atheromatous deposit. The popliteal pulse point is in the popliteal space, behind the knee.

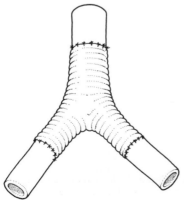

Figure 14. Aorto-iliac by-pass graft—'the trousergraft'.

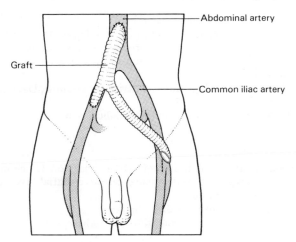

Figure 15. Aorta to left femoral artery and right common iliac artery by-pass using a synthetic (Dacron) graft.

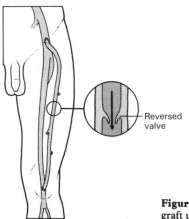

Figure 16. Femoral artery by-pass graft using the long saphenous vein.

Materials used for by-pass surgery
1 The patient's own long saphenous vein (Figure 16); however, this vein may be needed for coronary by-pass surgery later, bearing in mind that atherosclerosis is a degenerative and progressive disease.
2 Woven or knitted synthetic material, for example, Dacron (a polyester) (Figures 14 and 15).
3 Preserved, reinforced, human umbilical vein.

Investigation

The aim of surgery is to improve the arterial flow to the limb and before surgery is contemplated certain essential investigations will be carried out.
1 ECG: to determine cardiac function.
2 Measurement of arterial flow in both legs by Doppler flowmeter.
3 Saphenogram: to determine whether the saphenous vein is available as by-pass material, if required. This investigation is usually performed with a local anaesthetic.
4 Arteriogram: to determine the site and extent of the obstruction. This may involve a trans-lumbar approach and is carried out under a general anaesthetic.

Nursing activities following arteriogram
It is important to be aware that all forms of arteriogram carry a slight risk.
- Observe for signs of internal bleeding.
- Observe for bleeding from puncture site; apply a pressure dressing.
- Restrict the patient's activity for 24 hours following the investigation.
- Explain all the procedures to the patient, giving the reasons for the observations and for the restrictions.

Assessment on admission

Related nursing activities
- Does the patient experience pain in the buttock, thigh or calf? Is this pain in one or both legs?
- Is the pain present when exercising, and does it stop when resting? This is intermittent claudication.

- Is the temperature the same in both legs?
- Are there any trophic changes present: is the skin scaly, shiny, and hairless?
- Are pulses present (Figure 13)?
- Are there any gangrenous changes: namely, blackened, hard and dry skin? If infection is present the skin may be moist with pus present.

Nursing care of the patient undergoing arterial by-pass surgery

Identification of needs
- Relief of pain, alleviation of anxiety and resolution, if possible, of fears.
- Care of ischaemic limbs; heels are particularly vulnerable to pressure.
- Careful observation.

Related nursing activities—preoperative
- Pain may be present only at exercise and rest may bring relief, but more extensive disease may mean that pain is severe and present even at rest; it may also be worse during the long night hours. Paracetamol may be effective to ease mild discomfort but for severe pain which is continuous and psychologically debilitating, the patient will need a stronger analgesic such as dextromoramide 5 mg orally every four hours or oral dihydrocodeine 30–60 mg orally every four hours. Some relief may be obtained by elevating the head of the bed and the patient may wish to hang his legs over the side of the bed. Alcohol, for example whisky, may help to promote peripheral vascular dilatation and reduce anxiety. Night sedation will be helpful.
- Careful, consistent attention should be given to pressure areas, particularly to heels, sacral area and elbows. Sheepskins should always be used and the weight of bed linen should be kept off limbs by a bed-cradle; this will also allow free circulation of cool air. The danger of accidental trauma to ischaemic limbs cannot be overemphasized.
- Gangrenous areas should be kept clean and dry and toes should be separated where necessary. Bacterial infection may be treated with the appropriate antimicrobial drug.

- The presence of pulses should be determined and compared with those recorded on the initial assessment; the absence of a pulse previously felt should be immediately reported. The temperature of extremities should be recorded, together with any colour changes. Urinalysis should be carried out, as there is a strong association between peripheral vascular disease and diabetes mellitus.
- Clear explanations and support should be given to the patient and his relatives throughout.

Related nursing activities—postoperative
The prime nursing responsibility is the recognition of early signs of complications, specifically *reduction or cessation of blood flow* through the by-pass graft, indicating closure of the graft, *swelling,* indicating haematoma, or *haemorrhage* from the suture line.

- The colour and the temperature of the limb should be observed: it should be pink and warm and initially it may be warmer than the other leg. Sudden changes in colour or temperature should be reported immediately.
- Pulses should be present, specifically the dorsalis pedis and anterior tibial pulses (Figure 13). The popliteal pulse is more difficult to palpate and it is not usually necessary for the nurse to record its presence. This applies also to the femoral pulse, which is often under a groin incision. When pulses have been identified, they should be lightly marked in order that they may be located easily by any nurse who may be called upon to look after the patient. It will reduce the latter's anxiety and doubt if pulses are felt quickly and efficiently; to this end the legs should be exposed under the bed-cradle, free from bed linen, in the early stages. Any loss of pulses should be checked by another member of staff and reported immediately; it may mean that the graft has closed off and the patient needs to be returned to theatre at once for exploration and possible embolectomy (removal of the clot).
- Any oozing from the suture line, any sudden loss of blood through drainage tubes or systemic signs of bleeding should be reported immediately.

Continuing care
- The patient should be supported in a semi-upright position in order that deep-breathing exercises can be carried out and

gentle leg exercises performed. Analgesia should be given before physiotherapy, in order that the patient can cooperate effectively with the physiotherapist.

- Urine output should be observed, recorded and any diminution in output reported at once. In any operation in which the blood supply to the kidneys may have been disrupted, the possibility of renal failure cannot be ignored.
- Drainage tubes will be removed within 48 hours.
- Sutures will be removed from the groin after 7 days and from the abdomen after 10–14 days.
- Ambulation is usually encouraged on the third postoperative day and is limited to walking round the bed on the first day and increasing the distances daily.
- A late complication may be infection at the graft site, which could lead to rejection of the graft. For this reason it is customary for anti-microbial drugs to be prescribed, for example, flucloxacillin 500 mg four times a day for 10 days.

Future health considerations
- The patient should be advised to give up smoking; and counselling is often available for those who have difficulty in doing so.
- Exercise is encouraged; this may open up additional collateral circulation and enhance the prognosis for the by-pass graft.

Aortic aneurysm

The patient with a ruptured aortic aneurysm needs immediate surgery to repair the aorta or he will die. However if this major vessel is leaking as a result of an aneurysm but is not ruptured, a short delay may be possible. In this time the patient's general condition will be assessed, as will his cardiac function and the extent to which atherosclerotic changes are present throughout the vascular system. If the aneurysm is leaking retroperitoneally, this can be discerned from a CT (computerized tomography) scan.

Related nursing activities—preoperative
- Vital signs should be monitored constantly; the patient will be shocked but only minimal physical preparation may be possible (see p. 6).

- Analgesia should be given; severe back pain may be present.
- It is desirable to reduce anxiety; calm, competent handling, with explanations, will reassure both the patient and his relatives.

Related nursing activities—postoperative
Immediate nursing care should ideally be given on an intensive therapy unit, where continuous monitoring is possible. Blood loss may have been considerable during surgery and the adequacy of replacement must be assessed; careful observation and measurement by the nurse will contribute to this assessment. Renal function must be maintained. Complications may arise as a result of an inadequate circulating blood volume.

- Central venous pressure will be measured hourly; this is an indicator of circulating blood volume and should read between 3 and 10 cm H_2O (0.3–1.0 kPa), or as ordered by the surgeon responsible for the patient.
- Observation of pulse and blood pressure; a rapid pulse, a low blood pressure and cool clammy skin are signs that a further blood transfusion may be required.
- Observation for the presence of peripheral pulses and of the temperature and colour of lower limbs and feet. Thrombus formation with occlusion of vessels is possible after clamping of the aorta.
- Urine output should be measured hourly (the patient will be catheterized); an output of less than 30 ml per hour for two hours must be reported.
- Paralytic ileus will be present and the stomach should be kept empty by aspiration with a nasogastric tube.
- It is important to remember that the patient will not have been prepared for this major operation, which has a high mortality rate. He is usually elderly with pre-existing atherosclerosis. He may be confused and disorientated, having spent a long time anaesthetized and having undergone total blood replacement. He will need time to settle on return to the ward, with gentle mobilization while in bed and early ambulation together with lung expansion exercises.

Continuing care
- The inferior mesenteric artery which supplies the descending colon and sigmoid colon is clamped during surgery and a complication of this surgery is a necrotic bowel. The patient

may have diarrhoea which is bloody and persistent. The abdomen may be tender and distended. This is a potentially serious complication and it is important to observe and chart bowel action.

Future health considerations
- The patient should be encouraged to lead an active, normal life. As already stated there may be degenerative arterial disease present and it is considered desirable to reduce dietary intake of refined sugar and animal fats. Smoking should be actively discouraged.

Carotid stenosis

Atheromatous plaques may occur at the origin of the internal carotid artery and thrombus can form, partially occluding the vessel; this gives rise to transient ischaemic attacks. This thrombus may be surgically removed by carotid endarterectomy, through a long incision behind the angle of the jaw.

Related nursing activities—postoperative
- Close observation of recovery of consciousness, returning limb function and speech is necessary. There is a danger that thrombus may be dislodged and be carried into the cerebral circulation, causing a cerebrovascular accident.
- The incision is closed with clips; these are removed within 48 hours.

Future health considerations
- The patient may require bilateral endarterectomy; this will usually be carried out in stages, with about two months between the operations.

VENOUS SURGERY

The blood returns from the lower limbs to the right side of the heart via the inferior vena cava. There is a superficial and a deep system of veins, which are connected by other veins called perforators. The principal superficial vein of the leg is the long saphenous, which runs in the subcutaneous fat along the medial aspect of the limb, from the medial malleolus to groin, where it joins the femoral vein. The short saphenous vein runs in the lateral aspect to the knee, where it joins the popliteal vein behind the knee. The deep veins run with the arteries which bear the same names. All these veins contain valve-like structures, continuous with the endothelium, which prevent back-flow and, together with the contracting and releasing action of the calf muscle when exercised, promote venous return against gravity.

Varicose veins

The superficial vessels may become stretched, tortuous and distended (i.e. varicose) and their valves may fail to function efficiently. The incidence of this condition is ten times higher in females and there is also a familial tendency. This tendency may be exacerbated by occupational hazards, such as standing for long periods. Varicosities may first become apparent when intra-abdominal pressure is raised, for example in pregnancy, in chronic constipation or when a pelvic tumour is present. The symptoms are chiefly those of discomfort and aching in the lower limbs, mild ankle swelling at the end of the day and unsightly dilated vessels; the latter may be the principal reason for seeking medical advice. In the early stages these varicose veins may be treated by injecting them with a sclerosing agent. When the veins have been emptied by elevating the limb, the vein is injected and a firm elasticated bandage applied from toes to groin, with the limb still elevated. The injection will cause an inflammatory reaction within the vessel which will cause the endothelial lining of the vessel to adhere, closing the lumen. The patient is encouraged to exercise vigorously during the next eight weeks, walking long distances with the leg firmly bandaged, in order to encourage venous return via the deep vessels of the leg. However, surgery may ultimately be necessary.

Stripping and ligation of varicose veins

In this operation the superficial vein—the long or short saphenous vein—is stripped out by introducing a wire stripper distally; the vein is removed attached to the stripper. It may not be possible to remove the entire long saphenous vein through one incision and several small incisions may be made along the route of the vein. The vessel will be ligated where it meets the perforators and at the sapheno-femoral junction.

Related nursing activities—preoperative
- The skin over the vein to be stripped will be marked by the surgeon. The nurse responsible for the patient should ensure that the markings are intact when preparation for surgery is carried out.
- The groin should be shaved; this is an area which is sometimes forgotten.

Related nursing activities—postoperative
There is a danger of deep vein thrombosis after varicose vein surgery.
- The foot of the bed should be elevated throughout the postoperative period.
- Incision sites should be observed for oozing, particularly where multiple incisions have been made.
- The groin should be observed for any swelling or haematoma formation.
- It is of the utmost importance that the patient should be mobile as soon as possible and he should be encouraged to be ambulant within the first eight hours.
- The legs should be firmly supported when the patient is mobile and most surgeons will insist that elastic bandages are worn. Crêpe bandages are sufficient when resting on the bed. It is important that the patient is instructed in the bandaging technique, as it may be difficult to apply these when not practised in the skill. Tubi-grip supports are easier to apply and may be considered sufficient to promote venous return via the deep veins.
- The patient may have difficulty passing urine; early mobilization can often help to overcome this problem.

Continuing care
- The patient may be discharged after 48 hours, providing he has support at home.
- Any sutures will be removed at seven days after surgery. The incisions may have been closed with an adhesive strip, which may be removed when the legs are inspected, also at seven days.

Future health considerations
- Advice on diet should be given if the patient has a history of constipation.
- Support tights may also be suggested and the patient advised to avoid standing for long periods and to elevate the legs when sitting down.

Venous ulcers

These ulcers usually result from a disordered pattern of blood flow, arising from incompetence of the deep veins. There may be an earlier history of venous thrombosis with subsequent damage to valves at the affected site. The area normally involved is the lower third of the medial aspect of the lower leg. There are often eczematous skin changes and discolouration. Stasis of the circulation results in poor oxygenation and any minor trauma can result in a broken ulcerated area which does not heal. It is rarely painful but there may be discomfort.

Related nursing activities
It may be necessary to admit the patient if the ulcer has remained intractable over a long period.
- Bed rest is essential, with the foot of the bed elevated.
- The ulcer may be treated with a desloughing agent, at least daily, until clean. Antimicrobial drugs may be prescribed if the ulcer is infected.
- Once healing begins to take place, a paste bandage may be applied; this allows the patient to be mobile. The bandage will remain untouched for 14 days, after which the ulcer will be inspected and if necessary a fresh paste bandage applied. The bandage is impregnated with a therapeutic substance such as zinc or coal tar.
- It may be decided that a split skin graft is appropriate when the area is clean and once granulation tissue has appeared. (For care of a patient after a skin graft see p. 54.)

Continuing care
- Careful inspection of susceptible pressure areas should be regularly carried out and the patient should be encouraged to be as mobile as possible if bed rest continues.
- The skin around the ulcer is usually dry and scaly and should be regularly treated with arachis oil.

- Exercises to promote mobility of the toes and ankle joint should be practised regularly.

Future health considerations
- There is always the possibility that the ulcer will break down again and advice should be given about taking extreme care to avoid trauma. Restrictive clothing should be discouraged.

AMPUTATION OF A LOWER LIMB

Although the patient undergoing this operation may have suffered with intractable leg pain, both day and night, for a considerable period of time and the possibility of an amputation has been discussed, the final acceptance of this needs courage and considerable mental readjustment. Nursing care should be supportive, encouraging and realistic.

The aim of surgery is to fashion a functional, viable stump, which is able to support a prosthesis if possible. If the patient is old, frail and perhaps even bed-bound when at home, with only limited mobility, it may be more realistic to think of the future in terms of a wheelchair, rather than a prosthesis which will never be worn. The relatives who are concerned with the patient's future should be consulted and informed throughout.

Related nursing activities—preoperative
- The nurse responsible for the patient should be aware of facilities which will be needed and make arrangements accordingly. These may include: an appointment at the artificial limb fitting centre and with an occupational therapist who may liaise with the social services department of the local authority, if it is thought that the patient's house or flat may need future alteration or additions. The physiotherapist will make an important contribution, demonstrating postoperative positioning and muscle strengthening exercises.

Related nursing activities—postoperative
- Firm, even, stump bandaging to prevent the formation of oedema.
- Close observation of drainage tubes and the prevention, if possible, of a haematoma, which could result in wound infection and breakdown later.

- Close observation throughout for sudden and severe haemorrhage.
- The control of painful muscle spasm which may be present. This may be helped by gently but firmly applying pressure to keep the stump flat on the bed in the early stages; however, this is not always satisfactory or possible.
- Frequent, adequate analgesia in order to keep the patient as rested and free of anxiety as possible.

Continuing care
- The patient and his stump most be positioned correctly but comfortably, in order to prevent contracture. He should not sit on a sorbo ring. It is desirable that he should lie prone for regular short periods during the day in order to strengthen thigh muscles and prevent contracture. This is an uncomfortable position, which the elderly can tolerate for short periods only; the reasons for the position should be carefully explained.
- Early mobility should be encouraged and when the wound is sufficiently dry and healed the use of a pneumatic prosthesis is ideal, in order that the patient can quickly begin to adjust to a new centre of gravity when walking. If the amputation is through the knee or below the knee proprioception is not lost and early safe ambulation is possible. The physiotherapist is the best judge of progress in this respect.
- The suture line should be observed regularly and a firm bandage reapplied to the stump when necessary and as desired by the surgeon.
- Pain is often present for a considerable time after the stump has satisfactorily healed and every effort should be made to find the drug or combination of drugs which will be effective in relieving pain for the individual patient.

Future health considerations
- Every care should be taken of the remaining leg and advice offered on care of the heel when resting.
- Support, both social and financial, must be available in the community and all information should be made available to the patient and his relatives.

Further reading
Horton, R.E. (1980) *Vascular Surgery* London: Hodder & Stoughton.

5
Cardiac Surgery

Coronary artery by-pass

The incidence of coronary artery disease in Great Britain is not only one of the highest in the Western World but continues to rise; in the United States on the other hand, this trend has been reversed. In this country coronary artery surgery is carried out on some 50–100 patients per million of population, but in the United States surgery is resorted to in as many as 200–300 cases for every million of the population. It is suggested that some of the reasons for the decline in the incidence of the disease in the United States may be:

1   A dramatic reduction in cigarette smoking.
2   A growing awareness of the arterial problems which may be associated with excessive fat and sugar in the diet.
3   Effective health education which associates health with exercise.
4   Increased monitoring of blood pressure in the population generally.

The disease is primarily one of atheromatous damage in the vital coronary arteries, which supply the myocardium (Figure 17). The process involves hardening, distortion and consequent narrowing of the lumen of the vessel involved (Figure 12). The heart muscle is deprived of an adequate blood supply, its oxygen requirements cannot be met and the function of the heart, as a pump, begins to fail. The disease process is progressive and is manifested in its early stages by severe anginal pain and reduced exercise tolerance, which result in disabling changes in lifestyle.

Surgical procedures to revascularize the myocardium—*coronary artery by-pass operations*—owe much of their success to:

1   Advances in technological support available to the surgeon, such as extra-corporeal circulation (cardiopulmonary by-pass machines) (Figure 18).
2   Anaesthetic skills.
3   Courses available for training specialist nurses, skilled in immediate postoperative care.

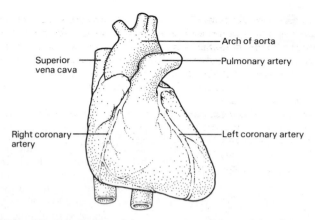

Figure 17. Distribution of the coronary arteries, supplying the myocardium.

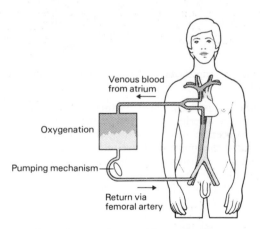

Figure 18. Cardiopulmonary by-pass (diagrammatic).

Cardiac surgery is considered, in the majority of centres, to be a team effort, in which the preoperative counselling, surgery, nursing care and long-term support are closely integrated. It is generally accepted that after by-pass surgery patients will be monitored away from the normal ward environment and receive intensive care for at least 24 hours. With increasing numbers of candidates for surgery and the necessity for cost-effectiveness in times of limited financial resources, patients will possibly be returning more quickly to the ward to which they were originally admitted. It is therefore the responsibility of nurses to be conversant with all aspects of the postoperative care that the patient may require.

It is not the intention here to explore the minutiae of intensive care nursing (see 'Further Reading'), but to convey to the student some of the knowledge which will help her to support the patient through preoperative preparation and the ensuing postoperative recovery period.

Materials used for by-pass surgery. The patient's own long saphenous vein is preferred; this vessel is able to withstand high pressure and has considerable tensile strength. This vein may not be available, for example because it has previously varicosed and been stripped, or it may not be suitable, if damaged by valvular disease, thrombosis or atherosclerosis. In such circumstances, the cephalic or basilic vein may be utilized, although there is an increased risk of occlusion when these vessels are used.

The aim of surgery is to by-pass arterial obstruction and improve circulation to the heart muscle by linking the aorta to a point distal to the obstruction (Figure 19). Most candidates for

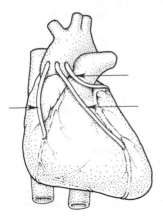

Figure 19. Possible coronary artery by-pass grafts (arrowed).

by-pass surgery are over 50 years old and it is important that some conditions which may be present are stabilized before surgery. These include:

a diabetes mellitus (generalized atheromatous changes are common in this disease)

b tooth decay or gum disease

c ulcerative conditions of ischaemic lower limbs

Essential investigations before cardiac surgery

1 ECG/echocardiogram

2 Dental examination

3 Cardiac catheterization and angiography. These are usually combined for coronary artery visualization; filling pressures in the chambers of the heart are measured by catheterization. The route by which the catheter is inserted may be:

a on the right side—via the basilic vein into the superior vena cava or via the femoral vein and inferior vena cava.

b on the left side— retrograde catheterization via the femoral artery.

The catheter is inserted under X-ray guidance and for angiography a radio-opaque substance is introduced.

Nursing activities before cardiac catheterization

- This is a sterile procedure; the entry site should be clean and, if necessary, shaved.
- Anaesthesia is not normally administered, but sedation, for example diazepam 10 mg intramuscularly, together with hyoscine 0.6 mg, may be ordered one hour before the procedure.
- An informed description of the procedure as well as the time and place, should always be given. A nurse from the ward should always accompany and remain with the patient.

Nursing activities following cardiac catheterization

This investigation may give rise to:

a arrhythmia

b bleeding with haematoma formation

c hypotension

Therefore the reasons for bed-rest after the investigation should be carefully explained.

- Observe for bleeding (check vital signs and the catheter insertion site).
- Measure blood pressure which may be lower than normal after catheterization because of the osmotic effect of the contrast medium used.
- Inform the patient of all activities and reiterate the reasons in order that confidence is maintained.

The patient should remain on bed-rest and activities should be restricted for between 12 and 24 hours, depending on the approach used for catheterization.

Nursing care of the patient undergoing cardiac surgery

Identification of needs
- Intensive psychological preparation. This is essential: every surgical procedure is special to the individual and his relatives, but heart surgery has a particular significance which has been enhanced by the universal interest aroused by the advent of heart and heart/lung transplantation.
- Educational preparation for long-term rehabilitation, changes in life-style, for example smoking habits and diet, and continuing medication.
- Clear precise information regarding the physical demands which will be made on the individual. This information should be reinforced by any informed member of staff who is able to form a relationship with the patient.

Related nursing activities—preoperative
- Psychological preparation starts immediately on admission, and many units have a set programme of group discussion and counselling, with literature available to reinforce the spoken word.
- The patient and his relatives will be fully informed, both in group discussion and individually, of the time of operation, about premedication and preoperative preparations and about the fact that he will be intubated and artificially ventilated for 8–24 hours after the operation.

- The importance of chest expansion exercises will be explained to him and he will receive instruction on breathing techniques which will reduce discomfort and maintain clear airways.
- Explanation will be given on the need for monitoring equipment, on the cannulas inserted for fluid replacement and measurement of vital signs and on the presence of a urinary catheter.
- The patient's worries about possible pain can be partially allayed by assurance regarding the regularity of analgesic administration. Supportive conversation and the company of patients who have experienced similar surgery is often very helpful.
- The bridge between the ward and the intensive care unit is of particular significance; the patient should be allowed to see all members of a collaborative team working towards a common goal—his well-being and recognition of him as an individual with his very personal fears and anxieties.
- Rest and sleep are essential; night sedation should be prescribed (for example, lorazepam 2 mg orally).
- Skin preparation depends on the surgeon's wishes, but usually consists of a complete body shave, antiseptic baths and special attention to hair, nails and oral hygiene.
- Prophylactic broad-spectrum antimicrobial drugs may be prescribed immediately prior to surgery.

Related nursing activities—postoperative
- Assessment of effective cardiovascular function after cardiopulmonary by-pass requires continuous monitoring of:
  1 Heart rate and rhythm.
  2 Mean arterial pressure—for control of bleeding.
  3 Central venous pressure—for accurate assessment of circulating blood volume.
  4 Left and right atrial pressures—for effective cardiac output.
  5 Peripheral pulses—for satisfactory peripheral circulation.
  6 Colour and temperature of skin.

- Observation for signs of restlessness and agitation, which together with other measurements may indicate tamponade, pain or respiratory distress.

- Care of the patient on assisted ventilation includes measurement of tidal volume and checking adequacy of air entry by auscultation at the bases and apices of the lungs. Removal of tracheal secretions and frequent estimation of arterial blood gases are necessary. When extubated, close observation must be continued for signs of respiratory difficulty or arrest.
- Control of pain will help the restless intubated patient, who may be 'fighting' the ventilator.
- Returning consciousness (which should be within one to two hours after surgery) can be assessed by signs of responsive, purposeful movement such as attempting to remove the endotracheal tube.
- Checks should be made on underwater-seal drainage tubes; tubes should be observed for movement of fluid and milked where necessary. Drainage tubes from leg incisions must be watched for excessive or sudden drainage and wound sites checked.
- Fluid balance and electrolyte replacement (especially potassium and sodium for effective cardiac contraction) must be assessed in conjunction with urinary output and all other physiological measurements.
- For possibly eight hours of this period, together with the time in theatre, nursing will be carried out with the patient in a supine position; a ripple mattress or similar device should be on the bed and working efficiently. Pressure areas must be examined as soon as the patient's condition is stable enough to allow turning.
- All activities should of course be explained to the patient throughout, quietly and gently.

Continuing care
When the patient is received back into the ward the use of monitoring equipment and other measures such as intravenous fluid replacement, chest drainage tubes and a urinary catheter will have been discontinued, and once the patient is settled emphasis should be on continuity of nursing care.
- Physical discomfort should be eliminated by careful assessment of analgesic requirements. Needs should be anticipated, rather than met when pain is apparent. An analgesic such as Paramol-118 (dihydrocodeine and paracetamol) one to two tablets orally every four hours, should be given. Pain can

often be relieved by reducing anxiety levels (see 'Further Reading'), for example by reassuring the patient that his chest incision is secure; if necessary, some support, for instance a pillow held tightly to the wound, will decrease the sternal instability which may be experienced after this operation when coughing. Deep-breathing and leg exercises should be encouraged, under the guidance of the physiotherapist.

- Positioning should be changed from side to side initially, to encourage lung expansion and removal of secretions.
- Rest should be encouraged, particularly at night, but exercise should be increased daily until, by the fifth postoperative day, the patient is able to climb stairs with supervision. Group exercise can be very successful and help to decrease apprehension.
- Observation of blood pressure, apex and radial pulse, temperature and respiration is continued until they are stabilized.
- Urinary output and weight are recorded daily.
- Wounds should be inspected and should be kept clean and dry; Sutures may be removed from five days postoperatively, according to the surgeon's requirements.
- Graduated support stockings are prescribed for the leg from which a vein has been removed. There may be a serous exudate from the distal portion of this incision and some ankle oedema, which usually resolves spontaneously.

Potential problems
- The patient may be sweating, anxious, nauseated and cold at the periphery. He may have a rapid pulse rate, an increase in weight and a low urine output. Treatment may be by administration of the inotropic drug digoxin (dose as instructed) and/or a diuretic such as Dyazide (triamterene and hydrochlorothiazide) (two tablets daily).
- Appetite may be poor, but this can be helped by cool nutritious fluids and light, easily digested, small meals.
- High anxiety levels may persist if psychological adjustment after surgery is not achieved and specialist help may be needed to resolve this problem.
- Close relatives sometimes perceive personality changes and need support throughout this anxious time.

Future health considerations
Specific advice relating to the following points should be available on discharge. They should be discussed in consultation with relatives.

1 Exercise. In the first three days exercise should consist of gentle walking and climbing stairs two or three times a day, progressing to walking outside, but not immediately after meals. From the second or third week activity should be increased to household chores, light gardening and so on.

2 Diet. Alcohol can be taken in moderation, weight should be controlled and smoking should be discouraged; adequate rest and sleep is essential.

3 Warfarin. Some patients are prescribed warfarin after surgery; this drug requires specific, written advice.

4 Sex. Advice regarding resumption of sexual relationships should be offered where appropriate.

5 Further advice. Information that ward advice continues to be available is a valuable source of psychological support.

Percutaneous transluminal coronary angioplasty

This was introduced in 1977; it involves the insertion of a balloon-tipped catheter via the femoral artery into the root of the aorta and thence through the obstructed coronary artery. The balloon is inflated, thus compressing recent atheroma, redistributing it within the wall of the vessel and reducing the obstruction of the lumen. This manoeuvre can be carried out during cardiac catheterization and may, in some circumstances, dispense with the necessity for surgery.

Valve replacement

The principles of care for valve replacement and coronary artery by-pass surgery are similar, but some points should be clarified.

Materials used
Replacements for the mitral and aortic valves are most commonly of two types:
Porcine (glutaraldehyde-treated) lateral-flow valves. These are effective replacements but have a disadvantage in that the recipient needs to be treated over a long period with anticoagulants;

these valves are, therefore, probably most appropriate when haematological monitoring is easily accessible for the patient.

Machine-made plastic/metal central-flow valves (Figure 20). These are tooled to an exceptionally high standard (1983 value approximately £1000), which is necessary for the work they will be called upon to do. This valve produces an audible 'clicking' sound which may initially be distracting but is soon tolerated.

Figure 20. Starr-Edwards valve.

Some surgeons now repair, rather than replace, the mitral valve initially, as the patient's own repaired valve is considered more effective than a prosthesis; however, replacement surgery may be required in the long term.

Further reading

Kelman, G.S. (1979) *Applied Cardiovascular Physiology*, 2nd edition. London: Butterworth.

Thompson, D.R. (1982) *Cardiac Nursing* (Nurses' Aid Series—Special Interest Text). London: Baillière Tindall.

6
Thoracic Surgery

SURGERY INVOLVING THE LUNGS AND RELATED STRUCTURES

Epidemiological trends have been reflected in thoracic surgery; pulmonary tuberculosis has been largely controlled, as a result of widespread screening programmes, improved nutrition and effective long-term chemotherapy, whereas the incidence of carcinoma of the bronchus and lung, associated with smoking and environmental factors, has increased. In the United Kingdom cancer of the lung accounts for 40% of male and 10% of female deaths from cancer, and while there is some evidence that the steep rate of rise in incidence in men is beginning to level off, in women it is still rising (see 'Further Reading'). As a result, surgical treatment for tuberculosis is rarely necessary, whereas surgical intervention for carcinoma of the lung is frequently being carried out in an attempt to prolong, and improve the quality of, life.

Investigations

Before surgery, which may mean *pneumonectomy* (removal of the whole lung) or *lobectomy* (part of the lung) (Figure 21), some investigations will be necessary:

1 Lung function tests—to assess the patient's ability to withstand the effects of anaesthetic and surgery.

2 X-rays, bronchograms and CT scans—for diagnostic purposes.

3 Endoscopic examination and biopsy—to identify pathological changes in the bronchial tree. The scope may be either (a) a rigid bronchoscope, for passage into the trachea and main bronchi, or (b) a flexible fibre-optic scope, which can be introduced into the bronchial segments and is able to visualize peripheral airways.

4 Thoracoscopy—a scope is introduced into the pleural space, under anaesthesia, to investigate for malignant disease of the

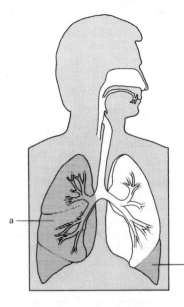

Figure 21. Areas removed in (a) right pneumonectomy and (b) left lower lobectomy.

pleura. After this procedure a pneumothorax will be present and nursing care will be necessary as for any patient with under-water-seal drainage tubes; this is described later in this chapter.
5   Pleural aspiration—the pleural space is cannulated and a specimen of effusion fluid obtained for histological examination.

Related nursing activities—before investigation
- A careful assessment should be made of the extent of any respiratory distress the patient may experience when positioned as for investigation. A patient admitted for investigation of dyspnoea, cough or sputum production may have difficulty holding a specific position for any length of time.
- Consideration should be given to the patient's ability to understand any instructions given during the investigation: he may be sedated but will not be anaesthetized for endoscopy. Can he hear and see? Does he normally wear a hearing aid or spectacles?
- Information must be given on those matters which will

directly affect post-investigation nursing care; for example, the nasal passages and upper respiratory tract may be anaesthetized and eating and drinking will not be safe until a swallowing reflex is re-established, so the first sips of water will be offered cautiously. Swallowing may be difficult and uncomfortable and there may be increased production of sputum, with slight blood-staining.

Related nursing activities—after investigation
- Bed rest should be maintained until the patient feels able to be up and about and a chest X-ray has been carried out.
- Observations must be made for signs of respiratory distress such as increased respiratory rate, noisy, obstructed breathing, a raised pulse rate, restlessness or haemoptysis; any of these would suggest trauma or pneumothorax.
- Frequent mouth washes should be offered, but fluids should not be given for at least four hours and then only water in small sips initially.

Nursing care of the patient undergoing surgery

Thoracotomy, an opening into the thorax (Figure 22) through the pleura, allows air to enter the pleural space (Figure 23). The pressure in the pleural space is normally negative, so entry of air will allow the lung tissue, which has retractile properties, to collapse; this is a pneumothorax. Any fluid or air which collects in the pleural space after surgery will need to be removed in order that the remaining lung tissue can re-expand and the pressure in the pleural space return to its normal negative state. Nursing care is centred on knowledge of this principle of surgical management.

Identification of needs
- Nursing procedures and the physiotherapist's skills must be coordinated, in order to maintain unobstructed airways throughout the procedure.

Related nursing activities—preoperative
- Smoking must be discouraged. This will be very difficult for a life-long smoker and restlessness and mood changes may

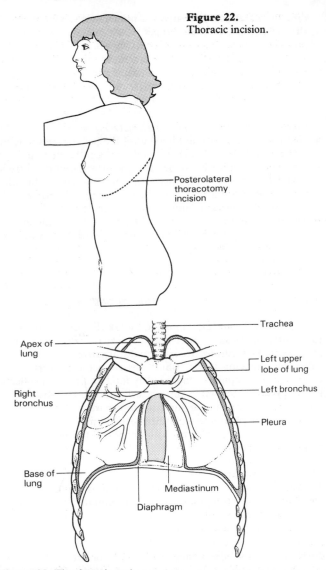

Figure 22. Thoracic incision.

Posterolateral thoracotomy incision

Trachea

Apex of lung

Left upper lobe of lung

Right bronchus

Left bronchus

Pleura

Base of lung

Mediastinum

Diaphragm

Figure 23. The thoracic cavity.

often be present. Some light physical tasks can sometimes distract attention from the need to smoke.

- Inhalations of compound benzoin tincture (Friars' Balsam) or menthol crystals will loosen secretions and help clear airways both before and after surgery.

- Chest expansion exercises involving the diaphragm should be demonstrated by the physiotherapist; the lung bases are rarely expanded in normal, everyday activities and secretions will consolidate at the base postoperatively unless actively removed by deep-breathing exercises, correct positioning and coughing. Once they have been demonstrated, it becomes a nursing responsibility to see that these exercises are continued effectively.

- An explanation regarding the helpful effect of oxygen administration and the correct use of a face-mask may lessen anxiety.

- A clear explanation regarding the reasons for drainage tubes in the pleural space should be given both to the patient and to his relatives, describing how he may assist and thus be involved in the management of these tubes; some information on the number of days they may be present is usually reassuring.

- The incision site should be shaved and the skin prepared as normally practised.

Related nursing activities—postoperative
- Observation must be made of respiratory rate and movements of the chest wall. Excessive sweating, restlessness, tachycardia and atrial fibrillation may all be indications of bronchial obstruction due to secretions after lobectomy.

- Deep breathing and effective coughing should be encouraged, and a comfortable position, well supported by sufficient pillows, to permit maximum chest expansion must be achieved. In the early stages it may be necessary to use suction to clear secretions, if breathing seems noisy and moist and the patient is not responsive enough to cooperate.

- Respiratory effort may best be facilitated—in pneumonectomy by positioning towards the affected side and in lobectomy towards the unaffected side.

Management of underwater-seal drainage
A complete understanding of the surgery performed together

with any written instructions regarding drainage tubes are essential before any nursing activities concerned with this aspect of care are undertaken.

Closed underwater-seal drainage prevents the collection of air, blood and serous exudate in the pleural space. The drainage apparatus acts as a one-way valve, allowing air and fluid to drain from the chest, while preventing air from entering the pleural space through the drainage tube (Figure 24). An *apical drain* is a single drainage tube placed near the top of the pleural space to remove air. A *basal drain* is a single drainage tube inserted into the base of the pleural space to drain fluid. Apical and basal drainage tubes may both be inserted; they may be attached to separate drainage bottles or joined by a Y-connection to a single drainage bottle.

After lobectomy the aim is to drain the cavity remaining, in order that the remaining lung tissue will expand and fill the

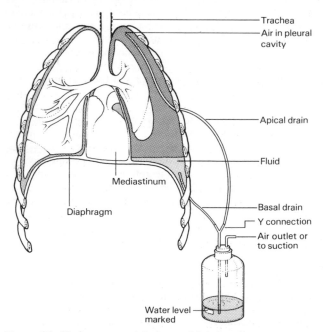

Figure 24. Underwater-seal drainage of the pleural space.

cavity. The tubes may be attached to suction apparatus. If this is so and there are two drainage tubes in situ, they should never both be directly attached to the suction source; instead a Y-connection should first join the two tubes (Figure 24).

The drainage bottles should always be below the level of the patient to prevent back-flow of drainage fluid into the space. The distal end of the tube inserted into the space should be below the level of water in the drainage bottle and be clear of its base.

After lobectomy the fluid within the tubing will be seen to 'swing'—rise on inspiration and fall on expiration—as the capacity of the cavity increases (inspiration) and decreases (expiration). Tubing should be milked of any obstruction to this swing.

The tubing should never be clamped during normal patient movement; clamping should only be necessary when tubing or drainage bottles are changed. The bottle should be changed daily and the tubing changed at least every two days. The amount of sterile water added to the bottle should be marked on it in order that an accurate measurement of drainage can be made.

After pneumonectomy drainage tubes, if inserted, will be clamped off permanently; they are usually removed at about 24 hours after surgery (after a check chest X-ray). This is to allow the cavity from which the lung has been removed to fill with exudate. Note that drainage tubing is never attached to suction apparatus after pneumonectomy.

The drainage tubing should be well supported as it emerges from the posterior chest wall; if it is allowed to hang unsupported it will drag, especially if clamps are attached, and may move with the patient's movement in the bed, rubbing the cut skin edges and being very uncomfortable. Redundant tubing is ineffective and only sufficient tubing to allow adequate movement is necessary. If the tubing is secured to the bed linen both the patient and the nurses should be aware of this.

Continuing care

- Effective analgesia administration should be planned to co-incide, if possible, with the physiotherapist's visit; effective chest expansion will not be possible if pain prevents the patient moving freely and means he is unable to concentrate or cooperate.

- Care should be given to the patient's mouth, especially when oral fluids are restricted and if oxygen is necessary.
- Gentle ambulation is to be encouraged even if drainage tubes are in position.
- After lobectomy, drainage tubes will be removed at about five days postoperatively (following daily X-ray checks for lung expansion and absence of air and fluid). This is a procedure to be undertaken by two nurses.
- Usually the tubing is sutured in position and a separate 'purse-string' suture is inserted; this will be tied as the tubing is removed. It is important that the patient is properly informed of what will be asked of him, the principle being to remove the tube when the pressure in the pleural space is as close to atmospheric pressure as possible; that is, at maximum inspiration. The manoeuvre should be performed quickly and smoothly and the suture tied firmly in a synchronized movement; a rehearsal is useful (Figure 25).

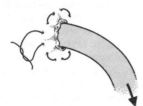

Figure 25. Purse-string chest drain suture, to be tied off when tube is removed.

- After this procedure, observations should be made for signs of respiratory distress, and a check X-ray will be carried out to ensure that the lung remains expanded; the importance of physiotherapy cannot be over-emphasized. The lung bases will be auscultated regularly and checked against X-ray pictures, and secretions will be removed by good positioning and effective coughing where necessary.
- The temperature should be recorded; a rise in temperature with blood-stained sputum and signs of mediastinal shift on X-ray could indicate a leak from the bronchial stump with a consequent bronchopleural fistula, especially after pneumonectomy. This may mean a return to theatre for reinsertion of drainage tubes. It is essential to nurse the patient on the

operated side prior to return to theatre as there is a danger of the fistula fluid spilling into the unaffected lung.

- A temperature rise may also indicate an infection in the space; if this happens a drainage catheter may sometimes need to be inserted so that the space can be irrigated as directed.

- Leaks and infections are, of course, set-backs for the patient and will delay his anticipated recovery; supportive, positive encouragement will be needed throughout and relatives should be kept informed. The patient will feel very unwell and in low spirits.

Empyema

Pus in the pleural space may need to be drained by insertion of a catheter or a more rigid wide-bore drainage tube and suction applied, if the condition is of a chronic nature and does not respond to chemotherapy.

Pneumothorax

This may be present as a result of incidents such as stabbing in a street fight or other violence and will be treated in the same manner, with underwater-seal drainage, as described above for planned surgical procedures. This condition may occur spontaneously.

TRACHEOSTOMY

It is sometimes necessary for a tracheostomy—a surgical opening into the trachea—to be performed; this may be an emergency procedure. Reasons for a tracheostomy include:

1 To reduce the dead air space. On inspiration 400 ml of air is inspired, of which 150 ml never reaches the alveoli but remains in the upper respiratory tract, where no gaseous exchange takes place. There are some circumstances where inspiratory effort might be beneficially conserved if a tracheostomy were present.

2 Where the upper respiratory tract is obstructed as a result of inflammation, for instance after ingestion of toxic fluids.

3 Where respiration has failed, for example in some neurological conditions such as damage to the recurrent laryngeal

nerve, Guillain–Barré syndrome or any other paralytic condition.
4 As a planned procedure in laryngectomy for malignant disease, where the trachea is brought to the surface as a permanent stoma.

The tracheostomy tube which will be inserted immediately after formation of the tracheostomy will usually be the Portex cuffed type (Figures 26 and 27), especially when intermittent positive pressure ventilation is to be employed, or where a paralytic condition is present. This ensures a close-fitting tube and prevents secretions from entering the bronchi. (Note that most

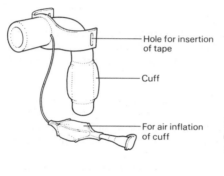

Hole for insertion of tape

Cuff

For air inflation of cuff

Figure 26. Cuffed (Portex) tracheostomy tube.

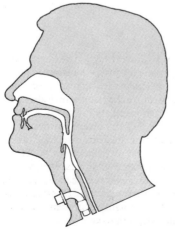

Figure 27. Tracheostomy tube in situ.

modern versions of this tube, once the cuff is inflated with air, do not require intermittent deflation, a precaution which has hitherto been necessary to prevent the necrosis of the wall of the trachea which can result from continuous pressure.)

Later a silver tracheostomy tube may be considered; a silver tracheostomy set consists of inner tube, outer tube and introducer. A speaking tube (such as the Negus) may be inserted; a valve at the outer opening permits air to enter but prevents its exit via the tube. Consequently, air flows over the vocal cords, allowing speech, something not normally possible in the presence of a tracheostomy.

In laryngectomy, where a permanent stoma is usually formed immediately, a cuffed Portex tube may be used initially, when haemorrhage is possible. However, there is little difficulty with re-insertion of a tube and the Portex tube is soon replaced by a silver tube. Speech, of course, is no longer possible if the larynx has been removed.

Identification of needs
- Communication. The aim is a comprehensive assessment of the patient's psychological readiness and his ability to assimilate information. The emphasis should be on the means through which he will be able to communicate his needs and how these can be met.
- Breathing. The mechanism of breathing via a tracheostomy and the part the patient can actually play in maintaining a clear airway should be explained.

Related nursing activities—preoperative
- Communication. This two-way process requires not only that the patient is given the basic equipment for the purpose—pad and pencil—and acquainted with any call system used, but that levels of understanding are recognized and language difficulties are overcome. The patient's relatives are of course integral to this process and should be fully informed of all procedures and given the opportunity to question and receive sympathetic support.
- Breathing. Suction apparatus should be explained and demonstrated and the patient allowed to handle suction catheters, oxygen masks and the humidifier. The presence of a mass of unexplained, often noisy, equipment can be distressing and cause unnecessary anxiety.

- Equipment. A brief description of reasons for careful, uncontaminated handling of equipment and removal of secretions
may be appropriate, but this may be more easily demonstrated postoperatively if the patient is to take part in his own
tracheostomy care and rehabilitation.

Some pre- and postoperative nursing activities will, of course,
depend on the reasons for the operation; for example, when a
tracheostomy is performed because positive pressure ventilation
is required for a longer period than is desirable via an endotracheal tube, although this may be a planned procedure, the
patient will not have been prepared in the conventional way and
postoperative care will need to be planned accordingly, taking
into account the psychological difficulties arising from the deficiency in preparation.

Another example is the patient with a malignant condition
requiring a permanent tracheostomy; he needs the skills of other
disciplines such as those of the speech therapist, the dietician or
the nutritionist. In addition, major plastic surgical procedures
may be necessary, for example pedicle grafting, which needs
special preparation and specific postoperative positioning and
nursing care. This will not be discussed here (see 'Further
Reading'). However, the general principles of nursing care and
the resultant activities can be described here.

Related nursing activities—postoperative
It is a nursing responsibility to maintain the adequacy of the
airway and to recognize signs of respiratory obstruction, such as
noisy breathing, poor colour, sweating, restlessness and tachycardia.

Tracheal suction. This should be carried out as often as necessary. This is an aseptic procedure in which a disposable soft
plastic or non-disposable rubber suction tube, usually size 12
(French gauge), is inserted via the tracheostomy to the level of
the carina; this stimulates the cough reflex and on withdrawal
secretions can be sucked out and removed. The catheter is
inserted, kinked at the connection and suction only applied as
the tube is withdrawn in a circular movement (Figure 28). The
tube should never be re-inserted: a new sterile catheter is used
each time suction is necessary. If the catheter is non-disposable, it

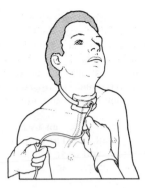

Figure 28. Suction of trachea on withdrawal of suction catheter, using a Y-connection.

should be soaked in a solution of sodium bicarbonate before re-autoclaving for re-use. It should be remembered that the patient cannot breathe whilst the catheter is inserted.

Tracheostomy care. The skin surface around the tracheostomy should be kept clean, dry and in the early stages may be covered. Secretions should never be allowed to collect and harden at the edges, causing soreness and discomfort, and thus providing the focus for a wound infection. Gauze dressings with unwoven edges should not be used; comfortable sterile plastic foam dressings can be obtained specifically for this purpose.

The tracheostomy tube should be secured with sterile cotton tapes, threaded through the side holes (Figure 28) and tied towards the side of the neck. Care should always be taken to ensure that these tapes are not confused with those which are often used on gowns worn by patients immediately on return from theatre.

If a silver tracheostomy tube is used, an additional tracheostomy tube and introducer should be kept at the bedside, together with a pair of tracheal dilators. In the early stages it may be difficult to re-insert a tracheostomy tube and in an emergency it may be necessary to maintain the patency of the airway by means of the dilators. The inner tube should be removed frequently (at least every four hours) and cleaned with a stiff brush under running water.

A plastic tube may be replaced by one of a smaller size or a silver tube; the first change of this tube is usually carried out by the medical staff.

- Positioning is important, to allow maximum chest expansion and the active coughing up and removal of secretions; the physiotherapist's invaluable knowledge here can mean that tracheal suction is less frequently needed.
- Oxygen and temperature-regulated humidity is usually prescribed; the humidity of the inspired air is important whilst the normal humidifying mechanism of the upper respiratory tract is not functioning.
- The opportunity to clean teeth and remove secretions by frequent mouthwashes should always be available. The mouth, lips and nose should be kept fresh, moist and clean and free from stale smells, which can be very unpleasant for the patient.
- Signs of fear and anxiety, for example, a tense anxious face with restless eye movement should be recognized; eye contact is crucial as a means of communication, and the anxious nurse can easily transmit lack of confidence to an already anxious patient. A cool encouraging hand can be reassuring and is often all that is needed to bring about relaxation.

Continuing care

It is important that all the equipment in use is cleaned, replacements provided and waste materials disposed of frequently; a clear, uncluttered working area is reassuring to the patient and is conducive to effective nursing care.

A temporary tracheostomy. Here the aim is eventual closure of the tracheostomy. Tracheal suction will decrease as the patient becomes more adept at removal of secretions by coughing. Chest expansion exercises remain of crucial importance and the early signs of a chest infection must be reported in order that possible antimicrobial treatment may be instituted.

The skin surrounding the tracheostomy area should continue to be kept clean, dry and if necessary protected from secretions.

When the patient's condition allows and a normal airway has been restored, especially if the patient has already been occluding the tube with his finger and attempting to speak or if a speaking tube has been in situ, the tracheostomy tube may be removed altogether or sealed with a dressing for a short period and the patient observed for signs of respiratory distress. Once the tube is removed the aperture will seal itself off within a few days.

Fluids are usually replaced intravenously immediately after a tracheostomy has been performed, and total parenteral nutrition or replacement via a fine-bore nasogastric tube may be necessary in a longer-term paralytic condition. When nutrition is given orally, semi-solids and thick fluids are usually desirable initially. Much reassurance may be needed in the early stages, as the patient is usually apprehensive and lacks confidence in his ability to eat and drink normally in the presence of a tracheostomy. Suction apparatus should be available and ready for use.

A permanent tracheostomy. Here the aim should be gradually to involve the patient, and if appropriate his relatives, in managing his care and to rehabilitate him to as near normal a lifestyle as possible. Tracheal suction should be demonstrated and supervised. The permanent stoma is usually formed from a portion of the trachea brought to the skin surface and sutured into position; there is normally no difficulty encountered in re-inserting the tube, and an inner tube is not necessary. A light dressing may be worn over the stoma during the day; this is compatible with everyday activity. The patient should never be in a position where water might enter the respiratory tract.

Drinking and eating will be managed as the patient's general condition allows: for instance, after laryngectomy there may be special nutritional requirements for which parenteral or nasogastric feeding may be desirable over a longer period, and the advice of the nurse nutritionist will be invaluable.

A planned progressive speech therapy programme for the patient undergoing laryngectomy may have been introduced even before surgery and will be instituted as soon as the patient is psychologically and physically ready to participate. This is only the beginning of an extensive rehabilitation programme which requires considerable fortitude on the part of the patient and his relatives, and sympathetic and positive support by the nursing staff to assist the long-term aims of the speech therapy team.

Further reading

Andreou, A. (1976) Underwater seal drainage, *Nursing Times* (27 June), pp. 1000–1001.
Royal College of Physicians (1983) *Smoking or Health* London: Pitman Medical.
Tiffany, R. (ed.) (1979) *Cancer Nursing* London: Faber.

7
Oral Surgery

Extraction of teeth

Many patients are nursed on surgical wards after total dental clearance, which may be a prerequisite for major cardiac surgery. The removal of wisdom teeth, which sometimes requires cutting into the gum margins and suturing after the extraction, often makes at least an overnight stay on a ward desirable. General principles of care are considered here.

Identification of needs
- Bleeding needs to be controlled.
- Mucous membranes must be kept clean, moist and free of infection.

Related nursing activities—postoperative
- Bleeding, if persistent, can be controlled by pressure; a moist swab, securely held, will normally be adequate. If the patient is conscious and responsive he will be able to do this himself, but the nurse must always be aware of, and take precautions against, the possibility of a swab being inhaled.
- Swallowed blood will make the patient feel nauseated and vomit; he should be encouraged to expectorate blood and saliva.
- Bleeding which continues should be reported.
- Antiseptic mouth washes should be offered frequently, once the possibility of further bleeding has been ruled out.
- Fluids should be encouraged as soon as possible, and appropriate food offered, compatible with the number of teeth remaining. If the patient is now edentulous (without teeth) he may be given a liquidized diet; almost every foodstuff can be reduced to liquid form. However, the muscular activities associated with chewing should be encouraged.
- The gums will be sore; soluble aspirin may be used as a gentle mouthwash if the patient's condition allows and if it has been prescribed. Any swelling present will usually resolve as muscular activity increases.

- Care should be taken to note any sutures which may have been inserted and need to be removed, at about three to five days.

Fixation of the jaw

The jaw may be wired:
1 to immobilize a fractured mandible
2 in some plastic, cosmetic procedures
3 as a method of weight reduction, to prevent the patient from eating.

Identification of needs
- The patient will be anxious and fearful, and require very careful psychological preparation.
- Communication methods must be established before operation as it will be virtually impossible for the patient to speak with a fixed jaw. The nurse should be aware of the problems associated with illiteracy.
- Dietary likes and dislikes must be discussed before surgery.

Related nursing activites—preoperative
- Everything which is possible must be quietly explained; the patient can breathe and can swallow; it is important to reinforce this knowledge as appropriate.
- If the patient feels nauseated after the jaw is fixed, this can be alleviated by:
  a slow concentrated breathing
  b intramuscular antiemetic injections (for example metoclopramide 10 mg, which stimulates gastric emptying)
  c the removal of sights and smells which may be causing the nausea
- Deep-breathing, chest-expansion exercises should be practised with the patient; excessive mucus and saliva production may cause a chest infection, which will complicate recovery.
- Suction apparatus must be available and explained to the patient; it is useful at this point to establish whether there are gaps between his teeth through which a suction catheter can be inserted.
- The patient should also be aware that there are wire cutters which will be immediately at hand if any difficulty should arise, but that this is a very rare occurrence.

Related nursing activities—postoperative
- As soon as the patient is conscious, reinforcement of assurances about breathing and swallowing is essential.
- Oral suction should be carried out as necessary.
- Moist lips and mucous membranes are important. Fluids will be administered intravenously initially.
- Antiemetic injections should be prescribed and administered.
- Discomfort and pain must be assessed and alleviated; it is important to report persistent jaw discomfort, which may be due to excessive pressure between upper and lower teeth and may require slackening of the wire by medical staff. Conversely, any movement of the jaw should be reported as the wires may need to be tightened.
- Soreness and chafing of the mucous membrane can often be relieved by dental wax placed around wires and over sore areas. Ulceration of the mucous membrane is a potential problem which can be avoided by careful examination.

Continuing care
- It is often possible for patients to achieve some degree of responsibility for their own mouth care and suction. A syringe can also be used for inserting feeds and for mouthwashes. As soon as it is possible to use a toothbrush, this should be encouraged. All equipment should be clean, dry and protected.
- Patients are often discharged with wiring in place; advice should be given on continuing care, as established during the stay in hospital. The support of a relative is essential; there should always be a telephone number available and access to advice, if needed.

8
Thyroid Surgery

The thyroid gland is situated in the lower part of the neck, anterior and lateral to the trachea. It consists of two lobes joined by an isthmus (Figure 29). Microscopically, epithelial cells are arranged around a central space containing colloid (Figure 30). The function of the gland, which is stimulated by hormones secreted by the anterior pituitary gland, is to utilize iodine obtained from the diet for the production of the thyroid hormones, thyroxine (tetra-iodothyronine/T_4) and tri-iodothyronine (T_3). These hormones are essential for:

1 the regulation of cellular metabolism
2 sensitization of beta-adrenergic receptors
3 cell growth

Goitre. Simple enlargement of the thyroid gland is a common condition in areas in which the diet or water is iodine-deficient.

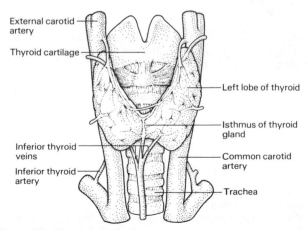

Figure 29. The thyroid gland.

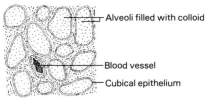
— Alveoli filled with colloid

— Blood vessel

— Cubical epithelium

Figure 30. The thyroid gland: microscopic structure.

Iodine may be filtered from water which has its source in mountainous or hilly regions before it reaches the population. As a result of the iodine deficiency, excessive amounts of thyroid-stimulating hormone are produced and colloid accumulates in the follicles. The increasing size of the gland can give rise to pressure symptoms such as dyspnoea, discomfort and stridor; neck veins will become engorged and the unsightly appearance will cause distress. Simple enlargement (hyperplasia) does not normally give rise to symptoms of hypersecretion (thyrotoxicosis) or hyposecretion (myxoedema), although long-term stimulation may result in a multi-nodular goitre.

Multi-nodular goitre. This developes as a result of disorganized glandular stimulation–episodes of hypersecretion alongside hyposecretion. In the early stages toxic symptoms may be present, but signs and symptoms of hyposecretion (myxoedema) may develop later.

Primary thyrotoxicosis. This may occur spontaneously or be triggered by puberty, pregnancy, infection or emotional stress (the condition is more often seen in the female).

Thyrotoxicosis and thyroidectomy

Thyrotoxicosis is a condition in which overactivity of the thyroid gland results in:
1 increase in cellular activity
2 increased beta-adrenergic receptor sensitivity
3 growth stimulation in childhood

The patient may experience many symptoms which can be related to these effects:
● She has a large appetite, but loses weight. She may have diarrhoea.

- She may sweat excessively and feel hot when those around her feel cold.
- She may feel nervous, irritable, excitable and easily stressed and be generally difficult to live with.
- She may be hyperactive, unable to relax, complain of headaches and have difficulty in sleeping.
- A fine hand tremor may develop.
- She may experience palpitations and be short of breath; on examination a tachycardia may be present with atrial fibrillation.
- She may have amenorrhoea.
- There may be signs of exophthalmos (abnormal protrusion of the eyeball).

These symptoms may be controlled by drugs, specifically *thiourea derivatives*, such as propylthiouracil, which prevent the formation of the thyroid hormones, and *beta-blocking agents*, such as propranolol, which will control atrial fibrillation and neurological symptoms. However, drug therapy will only control, not cure, the condition; up to seven-eighths of the gland may need to be surgically removed in order to bring about a cure.

Investigations

Blood specimens may be taken for serum assays of *protein-bound iodine* and *thyroxine (T_4)*.

Isotopes of iodine (^{131}I) (half-life eight days) and of technetium (^{99}Tc^m) (half-life six hours) may be administered (orally for iodine and intravenously for technetium) and the uptake of the substances measured by scanning. Visiting the nuclear medicine department can often arouse considerable anxiety and the skill of those working in the department is relied upon to dispel the fear associated with radioactivity. No special preparations are required prior to or after these investigations.

Nursing care of the patient undergoing sub-total thyroidectomy

Identification of needs

The patient must be euthyroid (without symptoms) before surgery is performed, so she may be admitted for control of her symptoms, described already, and her needs will be related to these symptoms.

Related nursing activities–preoperative
- Promotion of rest, quiet and freedom from emotional stress; night sedation may be prescribed.
- Provision of adequate nutritional requirements, the effectiveness of which may be measured by maintenance of a weight chart.
- Administration of prescribed drug therapy.
- Careful observation, particularly of the day- and night-time pulse rate, with apex/radial pulse recorded if fibrillation is present. However, it is customary for the patient to be treated before admission, where possible, and to require only the more immediate preparation prior to surgery.
- Description of the incision and the healing process. This should be offered in the course of general discussion with the patient. The incision is made taking the natural folds of the neck into consideration; when healing is completed the incision will barely be noticeable.

Related nursing activities–immediately preoperative
- Administration of prescribed drugs: iodide preparations (e.g. oral potassium iodide 180 mg daily) will make the gland smaller, firmer and less vascular. Night sedation is important.
- Provision of information regarding inspection of the vocal cords, an examination carried out both pre- and postoperatively to determine the mobility of the cords and the presence of any anomaly (a rare complication resulting from surgery could be damage to the cords, which may be irreversible and lead to litigation).
- Provision of information about the postoperative experiences:
  1 The patient will have to sit upright as soon as appropriate.
  2 There will be intravenous replacement of fluids.
  3 There will be drainage tubes from the incision.
  4 There will be clips or sutures and a pressure dressing.

Related nursing activities–postoperative
- Assessment of respiration: noisy breathing or stridor may indicate obstruction. Bleeding from the wound sites with

haematoma formation may produce pressure on the trachea with consequent narrowing of the airway; it may be necessary to remove clips or sutures to release the haematoma and then return the patient to theatre for resuturing.

- Observe for phonation difficulties; damage to the recurrent laryngeal nerve may immobilize the cords and obstruct the glottis.
- Observation for signs of tetany (muscular spasm resulting from reduction in serum calcium). Tetany may occur because of inadvertent removal of one or more parathyroid glands during the surgical procedure. The most obvious sign will be carpopedal spasm, and the patient may complain of paraesthesia–tingling, or 'pins and needles'–in toes and fingers and around the mouth and temporal region. This condition will necessitate administration, by a doctor, of intravenous calcium gluconate, with subsequent checking of serum calcium levels.
- Observation for signs of a thyrotoxic crisis. This is a rare occurrence, in which the pulse is rapid and irregular and the temperature is elevated, with increasing restlessness. This is thought to be the result of overspill of thyroxine into the circulation due to handling of the gland during the surgical procedure; it calls for urgent medical attention with prompt administration of oxygen and sedation. Digoxin and propranolol may have been administered prior to surgery and will be continued during this crisis.
- The patient must sit upright, well supported by pillows, as soon as her condition allows.
- The drainage tubes inserted in the incision will be observed and the contents of drainage bottles will be noted and the amounts charted, prior to removal of the drainage tubes (which will take place within the first 24 hours after surgery).
- Clips or sutures will be removed; usually alternate clips are removed within 24 hours and the remainder at 48 hours.
- Swallowing may be painful and fluids may be replaced intravenously for the first 12 hours, but oral fluids should be encouraged and frequent mouthwashes offered; aspirin gargles may also be helpful whilst discomfort persists.
- The pressure dressing should be removed within 24 hours.

Continuing care
- Early ambulation and gentle neck movements must be encouraged.

- The vocal cords will be examined again. Observation should be made of any difficulties that the patient may have in articulation; these should be recorded. A little hoarseness is normal immediately after surgery but should not persist.
- The incision can easily be disguised with appropriate clothing, and reassurance can be given that the healing process will eventually mean that the scar will be virtually invisible.

Future health considerations

Some patients may show signs, and develop symptoms, of undersecretion of the thyroid gland after surgery (hypothyroidism/myxoedema). This condition may be corrected by administration of oral thyroxine after assessment of serum thyroxine levels. It will be necessary to continue this medication for life. It is, however, a rare complication.

Signs of an undersecreting thyroid gland
1   General slowing down of the metabolic and mental processes.
2   Low temperature, blood pressure and pulse rate; the patient feels cold even in the hottest circumstances.
3   Thickened skin, thinning hair, and gruff voice.
4   Tiredness, weight gain and slow mental response.

Carcinoma of the thyroid gland

This is a relatively rare condition, which has been associated with radiotherapy treatment for tuberculosis, but this is no longer practised. Treatment is by total surgical removal or destruction of the gland by radiotherapy with iodine-131 and consequent chemotherapeutic support.

9
Abdominal Surgery

This chapter is concerned with surgery of the gastrointestinal tract and begins with a brief account of the tract and the abdominal cavity in which, with the exception of the oesophagus, it is contained (Figure 31).

The *gastrointestinal tract* is a muscular tube, approximately nine metres long from mouth to anus, lined with endothelial tissue, and structurally adapted for different functions along its length. Movement through the tube is peristaltic, with occasional mass movement, which produces a feeling of fullness in the rectum and a desire to defecate. Sphincteric control is exerted at certain junctures along the tract. The diameter of the lumen of the tube varies throughout and is capable of considerable expansion and distension, sufficient to allow a medium-sized coin, if swallowed, to be eventually uneventfully excreted. However, problems may arise in some instances, such as when a small bone which is sharp or of irregular shape is swallowed, when it may either become stuck within the lumen or perforate the wall of the tube. It is also not uncommon for whole segments of fibrous fruits, such as oranges, to remain undigested (particularly in those who have undergone gastric

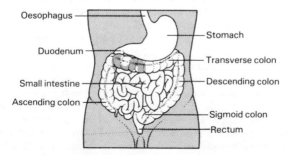

Figure 31. Structures within the abdominal cavity.

105

surgery); the lumen of the intestinal portion may become obstructed and surgical intervention may be required to alleviate the problem.

The *abdominal cavity* is bounded anteriorly and posteriorly by muscle and superiorly by the diaphragm; below, it is continuous with the pelvis. The cavity contains not only the gastrointestinal tract but also, among other structures, the liver, spleen, kidneys, ureters, abdominal aorta and vena cava.

The *peritoneum* is a serous membrane secreting a fluid derived from the adjacent interstitial fluid and containing water, electrolytes and other solutes. The *parietal peritoneum* lines the walls of the abdominal cavity, and the *visceral peritoneum* covers the organs (or viscera) within the cavity; it is closely adherent to each organ and its outer fibrous layer. The minimal space between the parietal and visceral layers contains serous fluid, which allows movement of one organ on another within the cavity.

The *omentum* is an apron-like double fold of peritoneum, which hangs down in front of the small intestine and ascends to the upper front border of the transverse colon. It is commonly filled with fat cells and can be surgically removed in the grossly obese individual. It is sometimes found, at laparotomy, to have walled-off areas of infection: by secreting serous fluid and wrapping itself around an inflammatory mass (resulting in, for example, an appendix abscess) it prevents the spread of infection into the peritoneal cavity and subsequent peritonitis.

The *mesentery* is a fan-shaped portion of peritoneum which is attached by its narrowest border (16 cm wide) to the posterior abdominal wall, completely enveloping the small intestine in its folds; at its widest it can be expanded to about six metres wide. Between the folds of the membrane run the blood vessels, nerves and lymphatic vessels to the small intestine.

The characteristics of abdominal pain as described by the patient are significant in clinical diagnosis. The gut is insensitive to stimuli such as cutting and burning but sensitive to tension on the mesentery, distension of its lumen, muscle spasm and ischaemia. These produce pain impulses which are carried by the sympathetic nerve supply to the viscera. The sympathetic nerves also supply the visceral layer of the peritoneum. The parietal layer of the peritoneum is supplied by the spinal nerves to overlying muscle and subcutaneous segments of the body wall.

Abdominal examination

The experienced clinician is often able to make a diagnosis from the following examination of the abdomen.

1 Observation of the skin. Striae may be present, indicating previous stretching during pregnancy or weight gain followed by loss. There may be assymetry or distension, visibly pulsating vessels and peristaltic waves.

2 Touch (palpation). This will determine areas of tenderness and confirm the appearance of rigidity of the muscular wall, which may be a result of either voluntary muscular contraction due to apprehension or involuntary muscular contraction (guarding), which may indicate underlying peritoneal irritation.

3 Percussion (gentle tapping of the area under examination). A hollow viscus emits a more resonant sound than a solid one and in this manner the presence of gases, fluid, tumours and enlargement of organs may be determined.

4 Listening. The abdominal cavity emits characteristic sounds of fluid and air in interphase, but these sounds may alter significantly; for example, there may be high tinkling sounds of exaggerated peristalsis in the presence of obstruction, and absence of normal sounds when mobility is inhibited by inflammation or paralytic ileus following surgery.

Identification of needs

The patient may experience varying degrees of pain, depending on the condition; pain and fear are inextricable and it may not be possible to provide analgesia until a diagnosis has been made (because signs and symptoms would be masked) and a systematic history, including details of significant symptoms, has been obtained from the patient.

Instructions about positioning for examination. The reasons for examination and questions asked must be given clearly and quietly, and every effort made to anticipate needs (for vomit bowl, urinal etc.) and help relaxation.

Related nursing activities
- There should be a good light.
- The patient should be supine, with one pillow, and his arms at his sides if possible, although certain types of pain (for example severe colic) may preclude this.

- The room should be quiet and privacy ensured; only the minimum amount of exposure is necessary for examination.
- Gentle, quiet breathing can be encouraged; this is often helpful as even the effort to concentrate on breathing can be psychologically therapeutic.
- Physical support may be necessary, for instance to sustain the left lateral position for rectal examination.
- The rectal orifice should always be left clean and dry after insertion of lubricating medium in rectal examination.
- There may sometimes be a communication gap (perhaps due to a language or cultural barrier) between clinician and client and, if invited, the nurse may often be helpful in this situation.
- If the possibility of immediate surgery exists it is important, in order to obtain the patient's cooperation, to explain the dangers of eating or drinking before administration of an anaesthetic. With severe pain and with reduced peristaltic activity within the gut, it is quite possible that the stomach will contain undigested food eaten several hours before the admission. (A written note of the time of the last meal taken will be useful.)
- Relevant observations, which will determine a base-line from which subsequent improvement or deterioration in the patient's condition can be assessed, should be carried out, charted and reported. The patient's own comments about any aspect of his condition should always be listened to with courtesy and he should be given time to describe symptoms in his own way; a chance, seemingly unimportant remark may, for example, save time and money by revealing that a proposed examination has already been carried out and records are in existence.

INVESTIGATIONS OF THE GASTROINTESTINAL TRACT

If the patient is admitted as an acute surgical emergency, investigations may be neither desirable nor possible, and surgery (a laparotomy) may be performed without investigations, perhaps with the exception of a plain abdominal X-ray. Principles of preparation before investigation will be discussed before describing specific emergency conditions.

Radiology
Plain abdominal X-ray. When the tract is obstructed, an erect abdominal X-ray will demonstrate fluid levels in the dilated loops of an obstructed bowel. An abdominal X-ray in the supine position may show gas under the diaphragm, which can result from a perforated viscus.

Barium contrast X-ray. Barium sulphate is a radio-opaque substance which in suspension can be administered orally or rectally and is used to visualize filling defects suggestive of ulceration or malignancy. Several techniques are used:
1 Barium meal: examination of the gastrointestinal tract from the upper oesophagus to the duodenal–jejunal junction.
2 Barium swallow: examination of the oesophagus, its peristaltic activity and the region of the gastro-oesophageal junction.
3 Follow-through: visualization of the small intestine, from the duodenum to the ileocaecal junction.
4 Barium enema: administration of barium rectally, visualizing the colon from the anus to the ileocaecal valve.
5 Single-contrast X-ray: distension of a cavity and delineation of the wall with barium.
6 Double-contrast X-ray: the cavity is partially filled with barium and the barium-coated walls distended by the insertion of gas.

Endoscopy
The *gastroduodenoscope*, a flexible, fibre-optic tube about 30 cm long, can be used for direct visualization of the mucosal surfaces of the gastrointestinal tract. Tissue biopsies and cells can be obtained for diagnostic purposes.
   The endoscope is increasingly used for therapeutic purposes, including laser therapy to seal bleeding vessels, removal of foreign bodies, oesophageal dilatation and insertion of a permanent oesophageal tube in order to maintain patency of the oesophagus when it has been partially occluded by tumour. Areas which may be visualized by the oral route are the oesophagus, the stomach, the duodenum and the first part of the jejunum. The ampulla of Vater, pancreatic duct and bile ducts can be visualized by the highly skilled technique of endoscopic retrograde cholecystopancreatography (ERCP) and it is possible

for small gallstones (revealed by T-tube cholangiogram after cholecystectomy) to be removed by this route.

The colonoscope, a fibre-optic scope 165–185 cm long, can be inserted, via the rectum, and entered via the ileocaecal valve into the distal portion (about 10.5 cm) of the ileum. This procedure is technically more difficult than gastroendoscopy and can take considerably longer to perform.

Other investigations
1   Computerized axial tomography (CT scanning). This investigation uses conventional X-rays to measure the density of abdominal structures; the information is processed by computer to give transverse cross-sectional pictures.
2   Ultrasound. This relies on the transmission and reflection of sound waves. It is a non-invasive technique in which a probe is placed in contact with the skin over the area to be examined.
3   Gastric function tests. These will rarely be performed, but can be used to determine the presence of secretions within the stomach, for example hydrochloric acid. The tests require the insertion of a nasogastric tube, the administration of a substance such as pentagastrin (a synthetic gastric stimulant) and the regular collection of aspirated stomach contents. However, gastric function is now more often the subject of haematological assay.
4   Many investigations are, of course, normal nursing functions; these include collection and testing of vomit, aspirate and urine for presence of blood and bile.
5   Collection of all faeces excreted may be required for assay of fat content where gastrointestinal symptoms are thought to be malabsorptive in origin.

Nursing care

Identification of needs
The following principles need to be remembered when considering nursing activities related to investigations.

● Any investigation which involves the insertion of a scope or the administration of a radio-opaque substance (which will assist in visualizing the tract) requires for its success that the tract be empty (unless specifically directed otherwise).
● Some investigations are invasive both physically and psychologically; therefore, adequate and careful preparation will

reduce the time required for the actual investigation and eliminate the possibility of the investigation having to be repeated.

- Investigations may be expensive in terms of both time and money.
- Information regarding the exact nature of the investigations, the reasons for it, the patient's contribution during the procedure and the after-effects, where any are to be expected, must be given clearly and repeated as frequently as the patient requires. It is incumbent on the nurse to inform the patient immediately of any changes in arrangements for investigation, particularly those which may mean anxious relatives cancelling long journeys.

Related nursing activities–before investigation
The gut may be emptied in many ways; preparation is dependent on (a) the custom usually followed in the X-ray department, and (b) the patient's general condition, nutritional status and age.

For radiological investigation and endoscopy of the upper gastrointestinal tract, it is usually sufficient for the patient to be without food or drink for about six hours or, if the examination is to be in the morning, for no breakfast to be given; an afternoon examination, however, may mean that breakfast can be taken. An exception would be an obstruction such as pyloric stenosis, which may delay gastric emptying and require gastric lavage before the investigation. Some 'follow-through' investigations may mean that the patient can return to the ward and eat normally until he is required for the next X-ray, but the ward needs to be informed if this is the case.

For investigation of the lower gastrointestinal tract, specifically the colon and rectum, the procedure is different; in order to achieve an empty bowel it is usual to restrict highly fibrous foods for a few days and to proceed to a high-fibre diet in the 24 hours prior to the investigation. It may also be necessary to perform a bowel washout, an enema or both. An oxyphenisatin (Veripaque) enema may be ordered immediately prior to the procedure.

Aperients such as castor oil may be prescribed until diarrhoea is present, and hypertonic solutions administered orally.

Preparation is often traumatic, raises anxiety levels considerably, and needs much nursing skill. Procedures should ideally be carried out in privacy, away from the bedside and with easy access to a lavatory and washing facilities.

Barium investigations are completed in the X-ray department. As the patient may have to respond to specific instructions concerning positioning, premedication is not normally prescribed. Endoscopy may be performed in an operating theatre or an area specifically designated for this purpose. Diazepam 5–10 mg is usually prescribed before the procedure, sometimes together with pethidine 25–50 mg i.m. and additional diazepam may be given intravenously during the investigation. Although the patient will respond to instruction during the investigation, it is rare for him to remember the procedure in detail on return to the ward.

Related nursing activities–after investigation

After barium investigation. Complications are rare, but it is necessary to ensure that all the barium is excreted.
- Where appropriate and prescribed, an aperient should be given.

After endoscopy
- Observation should be made for signs of bleeding from a traumatized mucosa.
- Nothing should be given orally until the patient is fully recovered, and, initially only water should be given. Fluid restriction applies also if a local anaesthetic spray has been administered.
- Any rise in pulse rate should be reported and the dangers of perforation should be uppermost in the mind when caring for the paient after this investigation.

Some patients may have ulcerating or inflammatory conditions such as ulcerative colitis or Crohn's disease, which may contraindicate preparation before investigation or even endoscopy itself; this is of course, at the discretion of the surgeon in consultation with the radiographer.

ACUTE ABDOMINAL EMERGENCIES

Perforation
Perforation may be caused when inflammation of the gastrointestinal tract occurs. This can result in the contents of this

hollow viscus spilling into the peritoneal cavity, causing peritonitis, which can also result from the spread of infection through the diseased wall of an organ such as gangrenous appendix. Some sources of perforation and peritonitis are:

a gastric or duodenal ulceration
b appendicitis
c diverticulitis
d Crohn's disease, ulcerative colitis
e malignancy
f stab wounds or accidental injury to the abdomen, which may, of course, perforate the gut.

Bleeding
A sudden, massive bleed from the gut may be due to:
1 Erosion of a vessel at the base of a gastric ulcer, acute erosive gastritis or carcinoma of the stomach.
2 Oesophageal varices (sudden rupture of vessels at the base of the oesophagus in portal hypertension).
3 Diverticular disease; a large quantity of bright red blood may be passed per rectum.

Bleeding, with the exception of oesophageal varices, may not be an acute surgical emergency, but will require replacement of lost blood by transfusion and investigation of the source of bleeding, before proceeding to surgery.

Obstruction
The gastrointestinal tract has already been described as a hollow secreting tube, propelling its contents onwards. Many of the conditions listed above, under 'Perforation', can give rise to obstruction, because inflammation within the walls of the tract may occlude its lumen, preventing absorption or excretion of its contents. The tract may also be obstructed mechanically by:
1 Volvulus (a twisting of the tube on its mesentery).
2 Adhesions (previous inflammatory responses, resulting in fibrous tissue formation sticking loops of intestine together) (Figure 32a).
3 Intussusception (spasmodic activity of the bowel, which pushes one portion inside a distal portion) (Figure 32b).
4 Ischaemic changes such as mesenteric thrombosis; these will reduce peristaltic activity and cause necrosis (death of tissue).
5 Paralytic ileus may be described as obstructive in its effects;

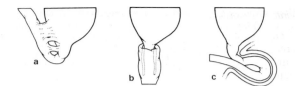

Figure 32. Some causes of intestinal obstruction: (a) adhesions, (b) intussusception, (c) strangulated hernia.

peristaltic activity is reduced in response to surgical handling and is a normal short-term physiological response to abdominal surgical intervention.

6 Hernia: pressure exerted on gut that has herniated into a confined space (for example the inguinal ring) will produce oedema, occlude venous return and arterial circulation, and result in gangrenous changes and intestinal obstruction (Figure 32c).

Principles of care in acute abdominal emergencies

Identification of needs

Relief of pain after diagnosis has been made. Pain associated with different conditions may manifest itself in various ways.

Pain resulting from perforation of a viscus (for example, in gastric ulcer) is severe, constant, epigastric and associated with shock, collapse and a rigid abdominal wall. As the peritonitis progresses bowel sounds may disappear.

Pain associated with acute appendicitis is central, abdominal and of a vague nature, but may localize in a few hours to become intense in the right iliac fossa, and be associated with vomiting and abdominal rigidity.

Pain associated with intestinal obstruction is colicky in nature with intermittent intense episodes, but background pain is always present; obstruction is associated with vomiting, dehydration, absolute constipation (there may have been earlier diarrhoea) and abdominal distension. Bowel sounds may be high and tinkling (obstructive) in character, but may disappear as obstruction worsens.

Maintenance of fluid and electrolyte balance

An empty stomach. This may prevent further vomiting and increasing distension in obstructive conditions, reduce irritation around a perforation and prevent further spillage into the peritoneum.

Related nursing activities

Observation. The decision to operate immediately will depend on the patient's general condition, and specific nursing observations will contribute to that decision. Careful observations should be made of:

- Pulse rate. This will be raised.
- Temperature. This will begin to rise if peritonitis is permitted to extend.
- Blood pressure. This may drop if circulatory fluids lost by vomiting or into the gut are not replaced intravenously as the patient becomes progressively more shocked.
- Vomit. This must be examined for the presence of bile, alterations in its colour, consistency or amount; as obstruction continues, vomit may change in character from containing undigested food to including bile, finally becoming stercoraceous (containing faeces). Blood may be present, either fresh red blood or brown granular (altered) blood, indicating partial digestion.
- Diarrhoea, or any flatus which may be passed. Melaena stools (containing blood) have a characteristic smell and a distinctive, tarry appearance.
- Excessive sweating and increasing signs of restlessness, or altered respiratory rate, which may indicate internal bleeding.
- Urine. This should be tested and measured routinely; the absence of urine output should be noted and reported as renal failure is a possibility.

Observations should be accurate and checked by a colleague if any doubt is present. Any significant change should be reported, but observations should always be carried out in conjunction with more obvious assessment, such as that of general appearance, skin colour and warmth, the patient's responsiveness and his ability to understand what is being asked. A nurse who is able to provide continuity of care may be the most suitable person to assess deterioration or improvement in a patient's general condition.

Pain relief. Pethidine 50–100 mg i.m. may be considered where pain is colicky in origin (that is, in obstruction), whereas morphine or its derivatives may be more effective where the pain results from inflammation. However, prescription of analgesia is of course at the discretion of the surgeon and should be administered as prescribed and as the patient's condition permits.

Fluid balance. Fluid and electrolytes will be replaced by the intravenous route; the amount will depend on fluid loss, electrolyte assay and haematocrit/packed cell volume (the volume of red cells in the blood, usually expressed as a percentage of the total blood volume). Three to four litres of fluid may be ordered initially over 24 hours, isotonic saline alternating with dextrose solution and additional potassium added where appropriate (see p. 15). A central venous pressure line may be introduced to assess the circulating blood volume more efficiently (see p. 18).

A nasogastric tube should be inserted, in order that the patient's stomach may be kept empty by aspiration, so preventing further fluid and electrolyte loss by vomiting and reducing the exhaustion associated with persistent vomiting (in obstruction).

Opportunity to rinse the mouth must always be available as oral fluid will not be permitted; gentle bathing of face and hands will refresh and comfort the patient.

Psychological care. Quiet, efficient, purposeful movement will reduce anxiety in this particularly trying time for an ill patient; clear, careful explanation should be offered before any procedure is attempted and careful consideration should be given to the merits of strict adherence to protocol which may not be in the best interests of the patient. It is a matter of fine judgement whether relatives should be present and the patient's wishes should be respected in this matter.

The patient needs rest, quiet and psychological security to promote physical well-being.

Specific care, before and after surgery, will be considered in the context of the following conditions.

THE STOMACH

Peptic ulcer

Peptic ulceration is a term normally used to describe both gastric ulcer and duodenal ulcers; both conditions involve ulceration of the mucosal wall (of the stomach and duodenum respectively) by the enzyme pepsin.

Features of *gastric ulceration* are:
- Age of onset usually over 50 years in males and over 60 in females.
- About four times more common in males than in females.
- More likely to affect semi-skilled and unskilled workers than professional workers.
- The ulceration occurs most commonly on the lesser curve of the stomach (Figure 33).
- Pain is associated with eating and may be relieved by vomiting; it is epigastric in origin.
- Weight loss is common.
- Malignant changes may occur.

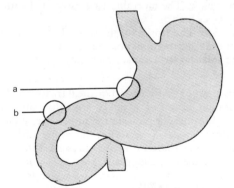

Figure 33. Common sites for peptic ulceration: (a) lesser-curve of stomach; (b) first part of duodenum (the duodenal cap).

Features of *duodenal ulceration* are:
- Age of onset usually less than 40 years in men and 50 in women.

- More common in men than in women.
- Four times more common in men than gastric ulceration.
- Occurs equally in all social classes.
- The ulceration occurs most commonly 2.5–5 cm from the duodenal cap (Figure 33), although pre-pyloric ulceration presents with similar symptoms.
- Onset of epigastric pain occurs two to three hours after eating, and may be relieved by eating, or drinking milk.
- Weight loss is not common.
- Malignant changes do not occur.

Peptic ulceration is associated with stress, anxiety and frustration, but there is no evidence to support the theory that these are developmental causes; the same may be said regarding personality type. However, smoking appears to be significant as an exacerbating factor. Although most ulcer sufferers have group O blood no genetic link has been established; there do appear to be familial tendencies, but these may relate to environmental factors.

Ulceration may be complicated by:
1 Perforation. This has been discussed previously (see p. 112).
2 Haemorrhage. The mortality rate associated with an acute bleed may be as high as 5%.
3 Penetration. The erosion of the ulcer through the wall without perforating the peritoneum, but producing inflammatory changes in adjacent structures, which may lead to fistula formation.

Symptoms may be persistent and medical treatment designed to heal ulceration may fail. The H_2 receptor site antagonists cimetidine (Tagamet) or renitidine (Zantac) are commonly prescribed. Barium meal X-rays and endoscopy with biopsy are performed before drug treatment is prescribed to rule out the possibility of malignant changes.

Surgery for peptic ulceration
A bleeding point can be visualized by gastroscopy (see p. 109). A perforated ulcer may simply be oversewn but may need further surgery at a later stage.

Gastric ulcer: Billroth type I partial gastrectomy (Figure 34). This removes the ulcer and preserves gastric–duodenal continuity; further ulceration rarely occurs.

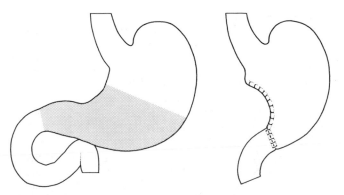

Figure 34. Partial gastrectomy with gastro-duodenal anastomosis (Billroth I gastrectomy). Left: portion of stomach removed; right: stomach and duodenum after surgery.

Duodenal ulcer: Polya type partial gastrectomy (Figure 35). The stomach is divided at the pylorus, the duodenal stump is sutured and the gastric remnant is anastomosed to a loop of the jejunum. The objective is to reduce the amount of acid secreted by the stomach (principally by cells in the antrum). Metabolic and mechanical complications are possible after this operation.

Truncal vagotomy and pyloroplasty. The vagus nerve is divided at the lower end of the oesophagus, and a drainage procedure performed to promote gastric emptying. The function of the vagus nerve is to stimulate gut motility and secretory activity; division of the nerve will therefore reduce motility and secretory activity. However, the reduction in gut motility requires that the pylorus be widened (pyloroplasty) or a further opening made into the jejunum (jejunostomy) to assist gastric emptying.

Selective vagotomy. A more selective vagotomy can be performed; in this the hepatic and coeliac branches are preserved and also the fibres running along the lesser curve to the antrum, thus allowing adequate gastric emptying (highly selective vagotomy). Only those fibres which affect parietal cell function (acid secretion) are dissected. The advantage of vagotomy, with or without pyloroplasty, is that there appear to be fewer metabolic problems; however, there is a possibility of recurrent ulceration.

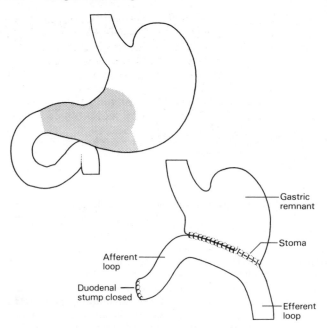

Figure 35. Polya type partial gastrectomy. Left: portion of stomach removed; right: stomach and duodenum after surgery.

Identification of needs
- Nutritional status needs careful assessment.
- A patient who has had an ulcer for a period of time may have been bleeding into the gut and will be anaemic; this will need to be rectified before an anaesthetic is administered (normal haemoglobin concentration 12–16 g/dl).

Related nursing activities–preoperative
- Every opportunity should be taken to encourage intake of nutritious food and fluid until restriction of oral intake is required. The stomach must, of course, be empty before operations on the gastrointestinal tract, but it is common practice for a nasogastric tube to be inserted when the patient is in the operating theatre, rather than the ward, unless there is evidence of pyloric stenosis and delayed

emptying, when gastric wash-outs will need to be performed preoperatively.

- A blood transfusion creates anxiety in many patients, the need for blood and the procedure for its transfusion should be carefully explained. Regular observations should be made whilst the transfusion is in progress (see p. 18).
- Information should be given regarding the need for drainage tubes postoperatively (for example the nasogastric tube) and for intravenous infusion.
- It is important to know whether the patient has been accustomed to taking analgesia for abdominal pain or indigestion; the dose may need to be adjusted upwards to meet immediate postoperative needs.
- Smoking must be discouraged tactfully, offering the reasons for this restriction and enlisting sympathetic support of fellow patients similarly deprived.

Related nursing activities–postoperative

Position. The patient should be positioned comfortably to allow chest expansion and he should be free of pain; if an antiemetic has been prescribed with the analgesia, it should be given, at least in the initial injection. Movement must be encouraged and susceptible areas observed for signs of undue pressure, especially in the undernourished patient.

Fluid balance and nasogastric intubation. Fluid and electrolyte intake must be balanced against output. Management will be according to electrolyte and haematocrit estimation; fluids will be replaced intravenously, taking into account blood and fluid loss during the operation and from any wound drainage.

It is necessary to have knowledge of the operation performed and consequently the exact position of the end of the nasogastric tube. It should be secured efficiently and comfortably, checking frequently that excessive sweat or grease on the skin have not made the strapping ineffective and that undue pressure is not being exerted on the nostril, which could cause ulceration or at least irritation. The nostrils should be frequently cleared of dried mucus, which collects around the tube. Times when the patient is to be aspirated should be clearly written on the recording chart.

The aspirate must be observed for fresh blood, which may be

present immediately on return from theatre (this should be reported: a tube positioned in the duodenum or jejunum will continue to produce large amounts of aspirate, even though bowel function has returned.

As bowel sounds return, indicating returning bowel function, aspirate will decrease; secretions will be absorbed from the gut, flatus will be passed and even though no food has been taken fluid intake may be sufficient to produce a bowel movement. Intravenous fluids will be decreased as oral fluid is increased and absorbed from the gut. On the surgeon's instructions intravenous infusion will be discontinued and normal fluid intake will be followed by a light diet, gradually increasing to a small normal diet.

While a nasogastric tube is in situ, frequent attention must be given to mouth care. Mouth breathing is inevitable; as well as mouthwashes, the patient must be encouraged to clean his teeth in the normal manner, especially after expectoration of sputum; lips should be kept moist.

Mobility. Progressive mobility is to be actively encouraged despite any attachments. Much encouragement may be needed to straighten up on the first walk and it is important, for this purpose, that effective analgesia is continued whenever the patient needs it: he may not ask for it despite his need.

Complications arising from surgery
Most operations are successful.

Billroth I gastrectomy. Complications are rare, but iron deficiency or vitamin B_{12} anaemia may develop.

Polya gastrectomy. Symptoms of nausea, giddiness and fainting may be experienced half to one hour after eating; this is thought to be a consequence of the osmotic effect of food entering the jejunum quickly. These symptoms tend to diminish with time. Patients should be advised to take small meals, frequently, and not to take fluids with food.

Vagotomy. Diarrhoea is sometimes severe but appears to be less of a problem after selective vagotomy. Symptomatic treatment may be necessary. Codeine phosphate may be prescribed.

Future health considerations
Stress can stimulate the production of gastric secretions and it may be helpful to be aware of those factors in a lifestyle which can have this effect.

Carcinoma of the stomach

This is a most serious condition with a poor prognosis, partly because the neoplasm may have reached a considerable size and have metastasized (to liver or brain) before signs or symptoms are evident. The disease is:

- more common in men than women.
- thought to be related to diet; although there is little evidence to support this, eating habits in different countries do seem to be related to the incidence of the disease.
- associated with loss of appetite, with consequent loss of weight.
- associated with difficulty in swallowing (dysphagia) and with regurgitation of food and the pain of 'indigestion'.

Depending on the site of the neoplasm, a partial, sub-total, or total gastrectomy may be performed (see p. 118). In the case of a growth at the cardia, it is sometimes possible to loop up jejunum or even the transverse colon and anastomose it to the oesophagus. As a palliative procedure, where gastrectomy is not possible, a gastrostomy or jejunostomy can be contemplated for nutritional purposes, and total parenteral nutrition is often considered, especially postoperatively when gross malnutrition can delay wound healing and recovery (see p. 20).

INTESTINAL SURGERY

For the general principles of immediate nursing care of the patient with an acute intestinal obstruction, see p. 114. The following is an account of diseases which may require resection of any portion of the lower part of the gastrointestinal tract. Any inflammatory process involving the wall of the gut may partially occlude its lumen.

The small intestine

Appendicitis

This is the most common surgical emergency. The appendix is a blind-ended tube, lined with mucous membrane, with a muscle structure similar to that of the caecum, which adjoins it; it is variable in size from 2 cm to 20 cm, averaging 9 cm, and is usually longer in the child than in the adult. It may occupy one of several positions, but always originates from the postero-medial wall of the caecum.

- The condition may develop from a faecolith which obstructs the lumen of the appendix.
- It may occur in any age group.
- Pain is initially experienced central abdominally, but localizes in the right iliac fossa.
- Nausea and vomiting may be present, and a history of constipation or diarrhoea may be elicited.
- The abdomen is tender and rigid.
- A tender mass in the right iliac fossa, with redness, swelling, fever and tachycardia, is indicative of an appendix abscess (as described on p. 106 when discussing the function of the omentum). The abscess may be drained and the appendix removed when the infection has dispersed, as a planned procedure.

Appendicectomy. An incision is made above the level of the anterior, superior iliac spine; the appendix is removed and the stump sutured. The cavity may be irrigated and a drainage tube inserted if any free fluid is discovered or peritonitis is evident.

Crohn's disease

Crohn's disease is a chronic inflammatory condition, which most commonly occurs in the terminal ileum, but can be present in any part of the gastrointestinal tract. The bowel becomes thickened, rubbery and oedematous; there is ulceration of the mucous membrane, with fibrosis and narrowing of the lumen of the tract. Loops of bowel may become adherent to each other and fistulas may be formed. There may be 'skip lesions'—interspersed with apparently healthy bowel.

- There is a history of repeated attacks of colicky pain with diarrhoea.
- The symptoms of this condition closely resemble those of appendicitis, and the diagnosis of Crohn's disease may only be established when the appendix is found to be normal.

Medical treatment is always the treatment of choice: resection of the diseased portion does not guarantee that the disease will not recur.

Mesenteric thrombosis

This is a very serious condition, potentially fatal. The mesenteric arteries may be occluded by thrombosis or atherosclerotic changes. An extensive part of the small intestine, which is supplied by these vessels, may undergo ischaemic changes, become gangrenous, and need to be resected.
- An early symptom may be pain after eating. Diagnosis may be confirmed by arteriography.

The colon

Ulcerative colitis

Ulcerative colitis is an inflammatory condition of the mucosa of the colon, rectum or both, with ulceration and oedema. The muscle layer is not involved, but fibrosis causes narrowing and rigidity of the bowel.
- This condition is characterized by frequent watery diarrhoea, sometimes bloody and containing mucus.
- It may be complicated by abscess formation, perforation, dehydration, malnutrition and anaemia.
- The patient with ulcerative colitis is usually nervous and anxious but the symptoms are sufficient in themselves to result in this characteristic disposition.

Treatment in the early stages is by conservative methods: anti-inflammatory drugs, both topical and orally, rest, rehydration, electrolyte replacement and nourishment. It is, however, considered unwise to allow ulcerative colitis to continue unabated for over ten years, as the indications are that it is a premalignant condition. The possibility of recurring symptoms means that consideration is given to surgical treatment before this time, as symptoms are frequently incompatible with a reasonable lifestyle. The surgery performed is usually total removal of the colon and the rectum (proctocolectomy), with formation of an ileostomy (see p. 130), which may be of the reservoir type.

Diverticulitis

This is a condition in which diverticula (pouches of mucous membrane, not supported by a muscle structure) retain static faecal matter. The mucosa undergoes inflammatory changes involving one diverticulum or a whole segment, usually of the sigmoid colon. Recurrent inflammatory episodes result in fibrosis—thickening and narrowing of the lumen. The wall may perforate.

- In acute diverticulitis there may be severe left iliac fossa pain, and the abdomen may be distended, with nausea and loss of appetite.
- The condition is very common in men; patients are usually overweight.
- There may be a history of constipation with flatulence and distension.
- Rarely, there will be a severe bleed in which a very large quantity of bright red blood is passed per rectum.

Conservative treatment for diverticulosis (generalized diverticula) is regulation of bowel function with the addition of dietary fibre to meals.

Surgery may consist of formation of a temporary colostomy, with further surgery to resect the colon when the acute inflammatory episode has subsided and the extent of the disease can be assessed.

Carcinoma of the colon

In the United Kingdom the incidence of carcinoma of the colon is second only to that of carcinoma of the bronchus. The site of the tumour is most commonly the sigmoid colon and at the recto-sigmoid junction (Figure 31).

- The carcinoma originates in the glandular cells of the mucosa (an adenocarcinoma) and on examination will be seen to be proliferative or ulcerative.

- Benign tumours (as occur in familial polyposis, an inherited condition in which there are multiple benign tumours) and ulcerative colitis predispose to carcinoma of the colon.
- It most commonly affects those over 50 years old.
- Males and females are equally vulnerable.
- The disease is characterized by changes in bowel habit, for example, episodes of diarrhoea alternating with constipation.
- There may be weight loss before appetite loss.
- There may be an abdominal lump which is palpable.
- There may be rectal bleeding or signs of anaemia.
- The onset may be slow and insidious.

The disease may spread: (a) by direct infiltration into an adjoining structure, (b) via the mesenteric lymph nodes, or (c) via the portal system to the liver. Treatment is by resection of the diseased portion of colon, where possible, and anastomosis. This may not be practicable (a) because of widespread infiltration or (b) where an adequate blood supply to a remobilized colon cannot be guaranteed. A colostomy will then become necessary.

Nursing care of the patient undergoing intestinal surgery

Identification of needs
All patients who undergo intestinal surgery need to be physically and mentally able to meet the demands made upon them before, during and after surgery.
- Mental preparedness is necessary for the possibility of altered body function (such as a colostomy or ileostomy), which will result in a change in body image.

Related nursing activities–preoperative
- Only the patient can come to terms with his altered body image, but skilled, informed support from nursing staff can create a positive environment.
- Physical and psychological preparation are not divisible; all physical preparation has a mental component and the least obvious psychological support may be conveyed when physical preparations are carried out. For the purposes of clarity, however, physical preparation is discussed separately.
- A careful assessment must be made by the clinician of additional fluid requirements, according to the patient's history,

symptoms, general appearance and haematological assay. The nurse will be responsible for fluid and blood replacement as instructed.

- Attention to nutritional status is desirable, if time allows, with the addition of vitamins and nourishing fluids, rather than tea or coffee. Opinions on the more specific aspects of intestinal surgery may differ between surgeons, but the general principle is that successful surgery, with minimal complications, is most likely if the gut is empty; consequently, foods high in dietary fibre such as vegetables, bran and pulses are restricted for about five days preoperatively, changing from this low-residue diet to fluid-only for the last 24 hours before surgery. Nothing will be offered for six hours prior to the time scheduled for the operation. It can be seen, therefore, that what is eaten must be nutritionally adequate. The dietician's advice should be sought.

- At the same time it is important that the bowel is properly prepared; again, this procedure varies from surgeon to surgeon. Some patients may be prepared by rectal wash-outs, and bowel preparations which destroy the gut flora are sometimes instilled per rectum or given orally. This procedure may reduce the activity of anaerobic bacteria and wound infection postoperatively.

  Note that in patients with inflammatory bowel disease such as ulcerative colitis or Crohn's disease bowel preparation may be contraindicated. If the patient has been taking steroid preparations previously, intramuscular hydrocortisone may be prescribed with the premedication and for postoperative administration.

- A shave is required according to accepted procedure (for example abdomen, pubic region and groins).

Related nursing activities–postoperative
- A careful assessment of pain must be made and adequate administration of analgesia, combined with an antiemetic, ensured.
- If the patient is free of pain he will be able to cooperate more effectively in chest expansion exercises and in increasing his mobility systematically over the early postoperative days, in order to reduce the possibility of a chest infection and the formation of venous thrombosis.
- It is common for a urinary catheter of the Foley type to be

inserted after intestinal surgery. If there is a catheter in situ, sterility must be maintained when urine is emptied from the drainage bag. Content will be measured and the amount recorded (on fluid balance chart). 60 ml of urine is normally produced per hour, but this may not be so immediately post-operatively (because of increased production of aldosterone and consequent increased retention of sodium and water); however, if the output is less than 30 ml over two hours, this should be reported. Catheters should be cared for aseptically, kept clean and free from secretions, and secured comfortably; a closed system should be maintained throughout.

- If a catheter has not been inserted, close observation should be made of urine output; urine retention is a complication after surgery involving the pelvic region. Male patients should have the opportunity to stand out of bed where possible, and access should be provided to a commode or a lavatory if the patient's condition allows.

Specific postoperative activities

Appendicectomy
- There is a high incidence of wound infection after appendicectomy, especially if the appendix has perforated. Therefore, close attention should be paid to the wound site for signs of redness and swelling with an accompanying rise in temperature and pulse rate; the patient may experience discomfort or painful throbbing.
- Management of a drainage tube, inserted if the appendix has perforated, includes:
  1 Maintenance of a vacuum at all times if drainage is of a vacuum type.
  2 Observation for and reporting of any excessive drainage.
  3 Careful attention to the drainage site: an aseptic procedure should be practised when dressings are changed if the drainage tube is of the corrugated type.
  4 Preservation of separate dressing sites if wound and drainage sites are separate incisions.

- Wound swabs may be taken for bacterial culture and antibiotic sensitivity testing if the wound is oozing or infection is obviously present.
- Antibiotics must be given as prescribed.

- It may be necessary to remove a suture prematurely if a haematoma has formed and needs to be evacuated.
- A long-term complication is the formation of adhesions, which may give rise to intestinal obstruction later (especially if an appendix abscess has been drained and, three to four months later, appendicectomy performed).

Ileostomy

When a total colectomy is performed, as surgical treatment for conditions such as ulcerative colitis, an ileostomy will be fashioned. The ileum is divided and the proximal portion (that section nearest to the functional part) brought to the surface of the abdominal wall as a spout (covered by mucous membrane) about 4 cm long. The contents of the ileum are fluid and contain proteolytic enzymes; moreover, the discharge is not under voluntary control and may occur without warning, so a collecting bag must be affixed to the abdominal wall to collect the fluid. A reservoir ileostomy may be formed (Kock's procedure), in which an internal bag or pouch is constructed. This pouch can be emptied several times a day, by passing a tube into it, thus obviating the necessity for an external appliance.

Colostomy

The colon is divided and its proximal portion is brought to the surface of the abdominal wall.

Temporary colostomy. A temporary colostomy may be fashioned (a) in an acute emergency such as an intestinal obstruction, (b) where there is a mass that is not immediately resectable, (c) where it is necessary to rest the colon, and (d) in conditions such as diverticular disease where there may be fistula formation. This involves bringing both the proximal and the distal loops of the colon to the surface, the latter as a defunctioning colostomy. There will therefore be two identifiable stomas emerging from one incision. Prior to closure of a temporary colostomy the distal loop may be washed out with water; a catheter is inserted into the stoma and the fluid is excreted per rectum if the distal portion of the colon is not obstructed.

Permanent colostomy. If the rectum or distal portion of bowel is totally removed a permanent colostomy is necessary. The contents and activity of a colostomy differ from those of an ileostomy. The contents are less fluid and the patient is capable of some control over function, especially if the colostomy is fashioned in the sigmoid colon. Control is largely established by regulating the food that is eaten in response to the effect that particular foodstuffs have on each individual. A method has been devised whereby a colostomy can be irrigated, once every two to three days. This will obviate the necessity for an external appliance, but certain home facilities are needed—time, space, privacy, water and a bathroom—and these are not always available to colostomy patients. The procedure is a simple one, involving an elevated bag of fluid attached to tubing which can control the flow of fluid into the stoma as a wash-out is undertaken.

Stoma care

Skin care. The skin must be kept dry at all times and protected from the excoriating alkaline contents of the gut by close-fitting stoma bags and meticulous attention to the care of the skin. A close watch must be kept for signs of allergic reaction to any of the appliances used; gentle cleaning with a hypoallergenic soap and careful drying of surrounding skin areas is essential. The peristomal skin protects against harmful invasion by chemical agents and bacteria, and must be kept intact.

The patient. Reference was made earlier to a supportive psychological environment and how it might be achieved. Honesty must prevail in this relationship, difficulties must be acknowledged and positive measures must be devised to overcome real or imagined difficulties. The following points are intrinsic to this.

Bowel contents smell; people in normal social interaction acknowledge only those smells which are considered pleasant and socially acceptable. Stoma bags are now highly sophisticated appliances and are fitted with filters, which allow the release of gases, but not odours. It is axiomatic that the nurse must not allow her face to reveal any personal distaste; the patient's main indicator of his social acceptability is the reaction of nursing staff.

- All equipment for bag changes should be assembled prior to the procedure.

- The procedure should be carried out expeditiously, and excreta removed promptly.
- Privacy should be maintained, preferably away from the bed area and near a lavatory where excreta may be disposed of.
- An aerosol spray may be appreciated.
- Intestinal gases can be absorbed by substances such as charcoal tablets.
- A stoma-therapist is invaluable and is often able to suggest methods which can overcome seemingly unsolvable problems.
- Very careful assessment should be made before suggesting involvement by relatives in this most intimate of needs.
- There are stoma associations, for both ileostomy and colostomy patients, which are able to provide support, particularly when the patient is ready to resume his place in society.

The question of control over the stoma needs to be discussed. As previously stated, an ileostomy cannot be controlled, but with judicious management of the times that meals are taken and the types of food eaten it is possible for many patients to achieve considerable success in controlling colostomy activity and even to dispense with an appliance altogether and to rely on a simple dressing over the stoma. This requires time, patience and the will to succeed.

Caecostomy

An opening into the caecum is performed, sometimes as a safety valve to preserve an anastomosis distal to it, or in the case of an acute obstruction of the colon. A catheter is inserted and the contents of the small intestine drained into a drainage bag or bottle. The precautions relating to skin protection are the same as for other stomas. When the catheter or other tubing is removed, the caecostomy incision usually closes spontaneously, without complication.

THE RECTUM AND ANUS

Carcinoma of the rectum

This carcinoma is usually ulcerating and friable and any bleeding per rectum should be treated with great suspicion. The clinician will always perform an examination per rectum when this symptom is disclosed, as most rectal carcinomas can be felt with a finger.

- Bleeding may be accompanied by mucus secretion.
- There may be local rectal pain.
- There will be anaemia and weight loss.
- There may be tenesmus (a persistent and painful desire to empty the rectum) when the presence of the tumour is experienced as the presence of faeces in the rectum.
- There may be colicky pain with abdominal distension and vomiting.

The advent of the surgical stapling gun has brought about considerable advances in the surgical treatment of rectal carcinoma; previously, tumours which were less than 10 cm from the anal margin necessitated removal of the whole of the rectum and the formation of a permanent colostomy (abdominoperineal excision of the rectum). It is now possible, in many cases, to resect the carcinoma successfully and to anastomose the colon to the rectum with metal staples, much nearer to the anal margin, thus removing the necessity for the formation of a colostomy.

Identification of needs
- The patient with a rectal carcinoma is usually anxious, thin, undernourished, anorectic, anaemic and dehydrated.

Nursing care of a patient undergoing abdominoperineal excision of rectum

Related nursing activities–preoperative
- This operation implies a permanent colostomy and requires skilled, informed nursing preparation before the operation.
- Nourishing foods and fluids must be encouraged, with the addition of vitamins and iron where prescribed.
- Diarrhoea can be a very discomforting symptom. Facility for washing and proximity of a lavatory are important; clean linen must always be available, along with the opportunity to wash out garments. This is sometimes a great source of distress and can be alleviated very easily with a little careful thought.

Related nursing activities–postoperative
Skilled nursing care is needed in this most important phase of major pelvic surgery.

- There is a perineal incision (plus an abdominal incision) which will be drained either by vacuum bottle or by Portex tube into a drainage bag. This tubing may be the source of considerable discomfort to the patient and every effort should be made to position him in such a way as to minimize this.

- Analgesia must be given, anticipating its need, when movement is to be encouraged.

- The perineal wound must be kept dry and clean. Sterile pads must be renewed frequently and kept in place by a T-bandage or elastic net pants. This area can easily become infected, which will lead to wound breakdown and considerably delay postoperative rehabilitation.

- A urinary catheter is always inserted for at least five days; it will be managed aseptically throughout.

- Fluids and electrolytes are always replaced intravenously; postoperative blood transfusion is usually necessary.

- The patient is taken slowly through the first 48 hours and on the second day is gently mobilized into a chair for a short period; it becomes uncomfortable to remain seated for any length of time whilst the perineal drainage tube remains in situ. This tube may be removed about five days after the operation.

Investigations of the anus and rectum

Any bleeding per rectum needs to be investigated and this may be done by digital examination, proctoscopy or sigmoidoscopy.

Digital examination. The patient is positioned left laterally (because the clinician's right index finger is most effectively used when the patient is in that position). The patient should be positioned as near to the edge of the bed as possible, with legs flexed; he must be encouraged to concentrate on rhythmical, deep breathing as this will help him to relax, prevent anal spasm and decrease discomfort as the investigation is undertaken. A lubricated gloved finger is advanced via the anus, where a fissure or abscess may be suggested by discomfort and spasm. The rectum can be examined for the presence of faeces, and the walls for the presence of polyps or tumours; it is possible to palpate the prostate gland in the male and the uterus and ovaries in the female.

Proctoscopy. The proctoscope is rigid and is inserted with an obturator in situ; the obturator is removed when the proctoscope is in position. A light source can be attached. The anal canal can be seen and the presence of haemorrhoids, fissures and polyps noted.

Sigmoidoscopy. The sigmoidoscopy is rigid, 25 cm long and 1.5 cm wide and has a bellows attachment which is used to inflate the rectum and colon as the scope is advanced. The lumen can be examined for the presence of blood, mucus and pus, and the mucosa can be examined for inflammatory changes, ulceration and so on. Biopsy forceps can be inserted and tissue specimens obtained for analysis.

Identification of needs
These investigations are an affront to the individual's dignity, a factor which must be considered at all times, and should be performed away from the bedside where possible.
- Explanation of each procedure must be given before it is undertaken.
- Sedation administered before the investigation will facilitate the procedure.
- A good light is necessary.
- Privacy must be maintained.
- The equipment–the sigmoidoscope and its light source–should be checked beforehand; anticipation of the clinician's needs will ensure that the investigation is carried out expeditiously.
- Any specimens obtained should be clearly labelled and correctly transported in the appropriate medium.
- Any investigation when tissue biopsies are taken, requires that careful observation is made for signs of bleeding or trauma to the wall of the rectal or sigmoid colon.

Other conditions of the rectum and anus

Haemorrhoids

Haemorrhoids (piles) are dilations of the veins beneath the skin of the anal canal; they may become congested when intra-abdominal pressure is raised, for instance when the patient strains at stool or is chronically constipated or in pregnancy. They may prolapse outside the anus, may become inflamed or thrombosed and may not return spontaneously to the rectum when the anal sphincter contracts.

- Haemorrhoids may bleed when faeces are passed and bright red blood on the lavatory paper is often the only disquieting symptom.

  Haemorrhoids are treated by ligation and excision of the dilated veins (haemorrhoidectomy) or by digital dilatation under general anaesthetic (Lord's procedure). In the latter procedure, fibrous tissue in the ano-rectal region is broken down, thus reducing obstruction to venous return. It is a minor, but effective, treatment and usually requires no more than 24 hours in hospital; specific instructions are required regarding diet and bowel habit, together with directions for inserting an anal dilator daily until a follow-up examination has been made as an outpatient.

Haemorrhoidectomy–identification of needs

- Haemorrhoidectomy is a painful experience, but one which tends to be treated with a certain ribaldry.
- Infection is a threat, since this is an area which is easily contaminated.
- A severe bleed is possible.

  a immediately postoperatively as a result of a slipped ligature

  b on or about the tenth day postoperatively as a result of infection

Haemorrhoidectomy–related nursing activities

- Adequate analgesia is imperative, preferably not with a morphine derivative such as codeine, as these have a tendency to cause constipation.
- A pack, which may have been inserted rectally, should be

removed, ideally in a warm bath, within 24 hours. Observation should be made thereafter for excessive oozing.

- Bowel action should be actively encouraged; to this end a normal diet, plus fruit and fluids, should be resumed as soon as appropriate. Aperients may be prescribed, for example Dorbanex 10 ml at night orally. Fear of pain on defaecation is a serious problem and every effort should be made to encourage the patient in this very normal activity. Once defaecation has been achieved, and provided analgesia is continued, this problem is resolved.

- Optimum hygiene must be promoted; a warm bath must be taken every time the patient has his bowels open and a fresh pad applied to the anal area.

- A digital examination is usually performed before the patient is allowed home.

- Bleeding per rectum may occur if infection is present; a raised temperature should not be disregarded.

Fissure-in-ano

A fissure-in-ano is a longitudinal crack in the anus, which opens every time the bowels are opened. Defaecation is very painful and constipation is common. Fissures rarely heal spontaneously. Treatment is dilatation of the anal sphincter under a general anaesthetic; the edges of the fissure may be excised to allow healing.

Fistula-in-ano

A fistula-in-ano is a connection between the lumen of the rectum or anus and the skin surface. Treatment is usually by laying open the fistula, followed by promotion of healing by granulation; the wound is lightly packed, the corner of a gauze square being sufficient for this purpose. The bowels may be confined for a few days. Frequent baths are encouraged.

Rectal prolapse

This is common in elderly women. The prolapsed rectum may become ulcerated and bleed. A band of polyvinyl sponge is inserted via a lower abdominal incision to surround the rectum and encourage fibrosis and fixation of the rectum. Alternatively, a purse-string suture may be inserted around the anus within the external sphincter layer. Proper attention to diet and bowel habit is imperative.

Perianal abscess

Perianal abscess is a localized infection in fatty tissue. The abscess may be incised and drained.

Pilonidal sinus (a nest of hair)

This is a small opening in the cleft behind the anus, probably congenital, which contains hair and is the focus of recurring infections with sinus formation. The sinuses may either be radically incised and left open to heal by granulation or be closed with primary suture. The latter procedure often requires at least two weeks of tedious bed-rest and the sinus may still eventually require laying open. Advances in wound treatment have led to increasing use of a variety of non-adherent, absorbent, conforming gel dressings, which can be inserted into a wound to promote healthy granulation and healing of these often extensive incisions.

THE GALLBLADDER

The function of the gallbladder is to concentrate and store bile, which is released through the common bile duct into the duodenum (Figure 36), under the influence of the hormone cholecystokinin, as part of the process of digestion of fats.

Gallstones are formed from cholesterol, mineral salts and bile pigments, sometimes around a septic focus; stones in the gallbladder (cholelithiasis) are said to occur in 20% of the population over the age of 40 years. They may be present in the bile ducts and a greatly enlarged stone can sometimes cause obstruction in the small intestine.

The gallbladder can become inflamed as a result of gallstones or without gallstones being present.

Cholecystitis

This may be a *subacute* condition, in which (a) there is a history of episodes of flatulence and abdominal discomfort and (b) the

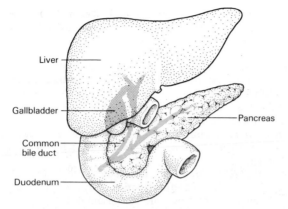

Figure 36. The gallbladder, biliary tract and related structures.

thought and smell of food is often difficult to tolerate (fatty dyspepsia). Alternatively it may be an *acute* condition, in which there is severe abdominal colic which may radiate to the right scapula, with tenderness in the right upper quadrant; there may be swelling in the gallbladder region. There may be jaundice, which is characterized by yellowing of the sclera, the mucosa and the skin. The pigment bilirubin, a breakdown product of red blood cells, is conjugated in the liver and excreted in the bile. If the biliary outlet is obstructed by a stone or inflammation there will be an excess of bile pigment in the plasma; this will be filtered by the kidney and will therefore be present in the urine (which will be dark in colour). Conversely, there will be a reduced amount of bilirubin in the faeces, which will therefore be clay-coloured.

The acute phase is usually treated symptomatically, and surgery (cholecystectomy) considered when the acute episode has abated and the diagnosis has been confirmed by investigations. Some surgeons will operate early if the diagnosis is uncertain or obstruction is suspected.

Identification of needs
- Pain and nausea must be relieved by quite large doses of analgesia (the patient is frequently of a large build and often

obese). Pethidine 100–150 mg i.m. every four hours as necessary, may be needed to bring effective relief, together with an antiemetic such as prochlorperazine 12.5 mg i.m. every four hours.

- The patient may be febrile and require intravenous fluid replacement, careful monitoring of fluid balance and recording of temperature.
- Antibiotics will be prescribed (penicillin is not excreted in bile and is therefore ineffective).
- Frequent refreshing washes are welcome, with particular attention to oral hygiene: saliva is reduced when dehydration is present.
- Bile salts present in the skin are a source of considerable irritation. In addition to careful attention to skin (keeping it dry and cool), an antihistamine–chlorpheniramine 4 mg orally three times a day–may be prescribed to lessen this discomfort.
- Patients with jaundice are often irritable and lethargic; these feelings should be acknowledged and supportive encouragement offered.
- The urine should be observed for the presence of bile and the faeces for its absence.
- Food low in fat will be offered as the acute episode subsides, and oral, non-milky fluids encouraged.

Investigations
1   Plain, abdominal X-rays (cholesterol stones are not opaque to X-rays).
2   White cell count (normal: $4-11 \times 10^9$/litre).
3   Liver function tests, for example serum bilirubin estimation and prothrombin levels (prothrombin is manufactured in the liver and obstruction of the biliary tree may lower its level in the plasma).
4   Ultrasound: the presence of gallstones in the biliary tree or gallbladder can be detected.
5   Oral cholecystogram. After administration of Telepaque (iopanoic acid) tablets:
    a   the gallbladder can be visualized on X-ray
    b   filling defects can be seen, which may indicate presence of stones
    c   failure to concentrate bile can be demonstrated
    d   delayed emptying can be detected after the oral administration of a fatty fluid mixture.

Cholecystectomy

Identification of needs
A tendency to obesity in these patients and the nature of the incision (right subcostal) mean that the patient may not expand his chest fully postoperatively; very careful preparation is needed to avoid this potential hazard. The services of the physiotherapist are essential.

Related nursing activities–preoperative
- The nature of the discomfort should be explained to the patient and the means for its relief outlined.
- Vitamin K 10 mg i.m. once a day for two days is sometimes prescribed if the patient is prothrombin-deficient.
- Smoking should be discouraged.

Related nursing activities–immediate postoperative
- The patient should be positioned to promote maximum chest expansion.
- A reluctance to expand the chest is understandable, if every deep intake produces discomfort. Analgesia should be judiciously administered, taking into account the activities in which the patient is to be engaged. An antiemetic should be given with the initial doses of analgesia, as vomiting is sometimes a troublesome postoperative symptom.
- A drainage tube, either vacuum drainage or a corrugated drain, will be inserted to drain the gallbladder bed (Figure 37) and will be removed after two to three days.

Exploration of the common bile duct
If a probe is inserted to explore the common bile duct during cholecystectomy there will be postoperative oedema, so a T-tube is inserted to maintain patency of the duct until the oedema subsides (Figure 37). This emerges through a separate incision onto the abdominal wall. The T-tube is of a small calibre and is made of pliable synthetic rubber or latex. A notch may be cut in the bar of the T, to facilitate removal. The tube will be sutured to the abdominal skin, and is long enough to coil and secure on the abdominal wall (before insertion into a drainage bag) to prevent inadvertent removal.

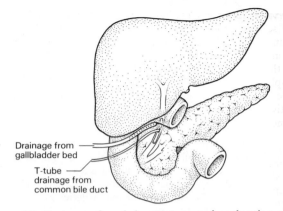

Drainage from
gallbladder bed

T-tube
drainage from
common bile duct

Figure 37. Drainage after cholecystectomy and exploration of the common bile duct.

Management of the T-tube
500–700 ml of bile is produced daily; the amount of bile draining through the T-tube will be an indicator of returning patency. (It should become less, but will not cease draining whilst a tube remains in place.)

Management varies, but the principle is to restrict drainage via the drainage tube, at about the fifth day, in order to test the patency of the duct. This is done by:

a raising the tube above the level of the abdomen, or
b clamping the tube completely, or
c clamping the tube for an increasing number of hours each day until, by the tenth day, the tube is totally clamped.

On about the tenth day a T-tube cholangiogram is performed: a radio-opaque dye is inserted via the tube, and the patency of the duct is assessed by X-ray. It is possible that the stones may not all have been removed at operation. It may be possible to remove a stone by endoscopic retrograde cholangiopancreatography and thus avoid further surgery.

Removal of the T-tube. This can provoke anxiety and administration of analgesia prior to the procedure is good practice. Removal is usually a simple process requiring only gentle traction, but on rare occasions it may be difficult; it is advisable on such occasions not to persist, but to seek medical advice.

Observation whilst the tube is clamped or elevated. Any abdominal discomfort should be noted; if the tube is unclamped the amount of bile drained immediately must be noted. Excessive, sudden drainage would indicate that oedema has not resolved, that there is some other obstruction within the lumen, for example another stone, or that bile is leaking into the perineum. If bile is passing into the gut normally, the urine will become negative for bile and be a normal colour; the stool will also resume its normal characteristics.

Observation after removal of the tube. The track formed by the tube may drain bile for about 24–36 hours; a dressing should be applied over the drainage site. Any drainage after this time must be reported. Any discomfort, pain or distension should be reported immediately as biliary peritonitis must be suspected. This is a potentially serious condition.

Increasing jaundice after a cholecystectomy may indicate an ascending infection and a potential bacteraemia.

Continuing care
A nutritionally sound diet should be advised—one which contains sufficient fat, but which will enable the patient to maintain a body weight commensurate with age and height. An appointment with a dietician should be arranged; long-standing dietary misconceptions can often be resolved.

THE PANCREAS

Investigations
1 Endoscopic retrograde cholangiopancreatography will aid diagnosis of pancreatic duct obstruction.
2 Ultrasound will demonstrate pancreatic disease.
3 CT scanning will identify an enlarged pancreas.

Pancreatitis

Pancreatitis is an inflammatory disease of the pancreas in which proteolytic enzymes leak into the gland and digest it.
● The disease is associated with alcoholism and disease of the biliary tree.
● Unlike biliary tract disease, which is more common in

females, pancreatitis is equally common in males and females.

- Pain, which is in the epigastric region, radiating to the back, is severe.
- The severity of the pain causes dyspnoea, nausea and vomiting.
- Pallor may be extreme; the patient may be collapsed and sweaty.
- Serum amylase levels may be raised above 1000 units/litre (normal: 70–300 units/litre).

Nursing activities will be as for an acute abdominal emergency (see p. 114):
- Intravenous fluid replacement
- Nasogastric suction
- Analgesia

Carcinoma of the head of the pancreas

Obstruction of the common bile duct may be due to extrinsic pressure caused by, for example, a carcinoma of the head of the pancreas. Surgery is usually palliative and aims to alleviate the distressing symptoms associated with severe and unremitting jaundice:
- Nausea, vomiting, anorexia and constipation.
- Skin irritation.
- Mental irritation and lethargy.

The obstruction may be relieved by anastomosing the jejunum to the gallbladder (cholecystojejunostomy), thus providing an outlet for the bile other than from the common bile duct to the duodenum. More extensive surgery may be undertaken, which involves the removal of most of the pancreas, the duodenum and the common bile duct. The remaining portion of the pancreas is anastomosed to the jejunum.

THE LIVER

Portal hypertension

Liver disease (cirrhosis) can obstruct the portal circulation in the liver; the resulting back pressure engorges the communicating vessels of the portal-venous system at the lower end of the

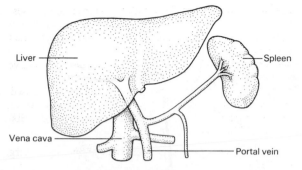

Figure 38. Portal circulation to the liver.

oesophagus, producing *oesophageal varices*. To overcome this serious problem, a surgical by-pass can be performed, either from the portal vein to inferior vena cava (portacaval shunt) (Figures 38 and 39) or from the splenic vein to the left renal vein, the spleen being removed.

Oesophageal varices can give rise to a sudden massive haematemesis; the emergency and life-saving action is to insert a tube into the oesophagus which, when inflated, will exert a pressure against the wall of the oesophagus, thus sealing the bleeding vessels. For this purpose a Sengstaken tube is used (Figure 40). When the patient's condition allows—that is, when lost blood has been replaced—one of the by-pass operations to reduce portal hypertension will be considered.

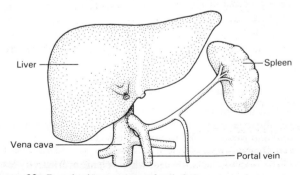

Figure 39. Portal vein anastomosed to inferior vena cava.

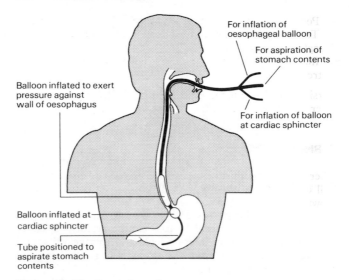

For inflation of
oesophageal balloon

For aspiration of
stomach contents

Balloon inflated to exert
pressure against
wall of oesophagus

For inflation of balloon
at cardiac sphincter

Balloon inflated at
cardiac sphincter

Tube positioned to
aspirate stomach
contents

Figure 40. The Sengstaken tube.

THE SPLEEN

This organ is situated in the left upper quadrant; it is a reservoir
for blood and part of the reticulo-endothelial system. Splenome-
galy (enlargement of the spleen) may occur in:
1 Infection
2 Congestion
3 Disease of the reticulo-endothelial system, for example
leukaemia and lymphadenoma (Hodgkin's disease).

Splenectomy (removal of the spleen)

The spleen may be removed in the following disorders:
1 Acholuric jaundice, a condition characterized by abnormal
fragility and rapid breakdown of red blood cells.
2 Lymphadenoma.
3 Thrombocytopenic purpura, when splenic overactivity leads
to excessive destruction of platelets.

4 Portal hypertension (described above).
5 Trauma, which may cause severe internal bleeding unless the splenic artery is ligated.
6 Inadvertent damage in abdominal operations such as gastrectomy.

Nursing activities will follow the principles already discussed for other major abdominal surgery.

HERNIAS

A hernia can be defined as the protrusion of a viscus through the wall of the cavity in which it is contained; potential sites are shown in Figure 41.

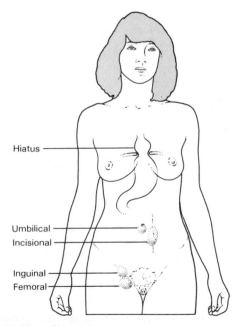

Figure 41. Sites of herniation.

Abdominal hernia

Inguinal hernia. In utero, the processus vaginalis, which descends through the inguinal canal into the scrotum with the descending testes in the male and with the round ligament of the uterus to the labia in the female, may fail to become obliterated and persist as an extension of the parietal peritoneum–a hernial sac (the inguinal sac: Figure 42). Any rise in pressure within the abdomen may push abdominal contents into this sac.

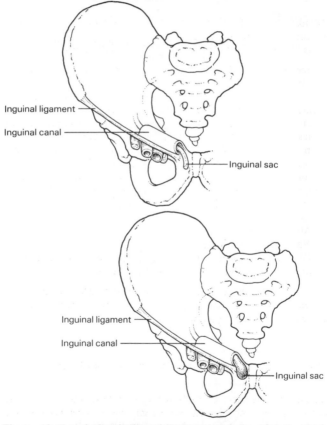

Inguinal ligament

Inguinal canal

Inguinal sac

Inguinal ligament

Inguinal canal

Inguinal sac

Figure 42. Top: the inguinal canal. Bottom: herniation of the inguinal sac.

Alternatively, this potential weakness in the groin region where the spermatic cord ascends may become a hernia later in life if abdominal pressure increases, owing to, for example:

a occupational hazard (the need to lift heavy and cumbersome weights)

b chronic respiratory disorder where there is a persistent cough

c constipation, resulting in straining at stool

d prostatic problems

Femoral hernia. Similarly, peritoneum and gut contents may herniate through the femoral canal, which opens into the groin. This hernia is more common in females than in males.

A hernia is described as *reducible* if the sac contents can be gently manipulated, by the doctor, into the abdominal cavity. It is said to be *irreducible* if the contents of the sac cannot be returned. An irreducible hernia is described as *incarcerated* when the gut cannot be returned, as a result of inflammation or adhesions, but its blood supply is not obstructed.

In a *strangulated* hernia the blood supply to gut contents within the sac is cut off, usually at the neck of the sac, as a result of compression (Figure 32); the bowel will become obstructed, gangrenous changes will occur and peritonitis becomes life-threatening. There will be:

- Colicky pain
- Abdominal distension
- Nausea and vomiting
- Obstructive bowel sounds initially, but progressing to absence of sounds if peritonitis supervenes.

A strangulated hernia must therefore be treated as an acute surgical emergency. If the gut remains viable, it is returned to the cavity. If not, a resection is performed.

Repair of a groin hernia (herniorrhaphy) as a planned procedure

The hernial sac may be mobilized, its contents returned to the cavity, the sac tied off and excess removed. Some surgeons may insert a synthetic mesh prosthesis to reinforce the deepest layer of the abdominal wall at the potential sites of recurrence.

Identification of needs

The patient will have been pronounced fit to undergo general anaesthesia, but if there is a history of a chronic respiratory disorder special attention will need to be given to this aspect of nursing care. (This procedure is sometimes performed under epidural anaesthesia, if the patient is not suitable for general anaesthesia.)

Related nursing activities–preoperative

- Chest expansion exercises and effective coughing techniques must be carefully explained. The services of the physiotherapist will be invaluable.
- Smoking must be discouraged.
- Careful shaving of both groin areas is desirable.
- Great discomfort may be caused postoperatively if the bowel is full; suppositories should be offered the evening before surgery.
- Care must be taken to ensure that the patient is aware of the need to have an empty bladder before a premedication is administered.

Related nursing activities–postoperative

- As soon as the patient is able to respond effectively, supported by adequate postoperative analgesia, attention must be given to comfortable positioning for maximum chest expansion, deep breathing and expectoration.
- Early mobility must be actively encouraged, unless there are specific reasons why this may not be so. Mobility may be a little delayed if the patient has a history of recurrent hernia, but this will be dependent on the surgeon's wishes.
- There are often micturition difficulties, which may be alleviated by standing out of bed with a urinal or by use of a commode; even more effectively, the privacy of the lavatory may be all that is needed. It will be wise to stay within calling distance, to offer support if it is necessary.
- If urine has not been passed within 12 hours, the insertion of a catheter may be necessary. If there is a history of prostatic symptoms, investigation of the prostate gland will be carried out or further surgery considered when the patient has recovered from his present surgery.
- The wound site must be observed for haematoma formation,

which may complicate postoperative recovery; a pyrexia may confirm its presence. It may be necessary to remove a suture to release tension on the suture line (if instructed), or a member of the medical staff may aspirate the haematoma by means of a syringe and an injection needle.

- If infection is present antibiotics may be prescribed after culture of the bacteria present and determination of the sensitivity of the organism to specific drugs.
- It is common practice to discharge the patient early after repair of an uncomplicated hernia, and arrangements will be made, according to specific hospital policy, for subsequent removal of sutures.
- The surgeon may advise the use of a scrotal support until the patient has fully recovered and the wound fully healed.

Advice on discharge

- Lifting of heavy objects is discouraged, at least until a follow-up appointment has been kept; however, if this is an occupational hazard it may be difficult to avoid once the patient has returned to his work (in about one month). Advice and written hints, which will demonstrate good lifting techniques and minimize the risk of hernia, should be available. Sedentary workers can often return to their employment two weeks after discharge.
- If smoking was successfully discontinued, friendly encouragement and reinforcement of this achievement should be offered.

Incisional hernia

If the abdominal wall has been weakened by a surgical incision or trauma, the contents of the abdominal cavity may herniate through the incision. The principles described for nursing care of the patient undergoing surgery for inguinal and femoral hernias apply. Additionally:

- The patient is frequently obese and will need support and advice on following a diet sufficient for his needs but aimed at reducing excess weight.
- A corset may be worn postoperatively to support the repair.

Intestinal obstruction can occur.

Hiatus hernia

A portion of the stomach herniates into the thorax through the oesophageal opening of the diaphragm. This is a common disorder associated with a short oesophagus in young babies and with obesity in the elderly. It may be aggravated by anything which raises intra-abdominal pressure. Symptoms, which are not always present, are:

- Heartburn, a retrosternal burning pain caused by a reflux of acid gastric fluid into the unprotected oesophagus
- Bleeding, leading to anaemia
- Dysphagia due to fibrosis

When other diagnoses have been excluded, by investigation, an abdominal or a thoracic approach may be used to repair the defect. Principles of nursing care must be directed towards the approach used.

Related nursing activities
The position of choice for the patient admitted with a hiatus hernia is the upright, well-supported, sitting position at all times, both sleeping and waking. The head of the bed should be elevated and stooping should be avoided. There is normally a pressure difference between the oesophagus and stomach; the pressure in the stomach tends to be lower than that in the oesophagus when sitting or standing but becomes greater when lying flat. Therefore, the upright position prevents regurgitation in hiatus hernia.

Further reading

Allen, D. (1977) Complications of T-tube drainage of the common bile duct. *Nursing Times* (18 August).

Breckman, B. (1978) Rundown on stoma problems. *Journal of Community Nursing*, **1** (11), 4.

Browse, N. (1978) *An Introduction to Symptoms and Signs of Surgical Disease* London: Edward Arnold.

Ellison Nash, D.F. (1980) *Surgery for Nurses and Allied Professions* London: Edward Arnold.

Goligher, J.C. (1977) The continent reservoir ileostomy. *Nursing Times* (31 March) pp. 447–449.

Johns, C. (1978) Formation of a continent ileostomy. *Nursing Times* (9 March) p. 396–400.

Roberts, A. (1981) Systems of Life No. 76. (Systems and Signs) Digestive System 2: Abdomen–Inspection. *Nursing Times* (April 2).

Roberts, A. (1981) Systems of Life No. 77. Digestive System 3: Abdomen–Palpation, Percussion. *Nursing Times* (April 30).

Roberts, A. (1981) Systems of Life No. 78. Digestive System 4: Anus and Rectum. *Nursing Times* (June 4).

Roberts, A. (1981) Systems of Life No. 79. Digestive System 5: The Acute Abdomen. *Nursing Times* (July 1).

Tinckler, L.F. (1978) The surgery of groin hernia. *Nursing Times* (14 September).

10
Urinary Tract Surgery

The urinary tract consists of the kidneys, the ureters, the bladder and the urethra (Figure 43). Urine is produced in the kidney and transported via the ureters to the bladder, where it is stored until it can be conveniently excreted via the urethra. Obstruction to the flow of urine can create pressure above the obstruction, which will be transmitted back to the kidney substance, interfering with glomerular filtration and causing renal failure if not relieved. Causes of obstruction of the tract include:

a   Renal calculi (stones)
b   Tumours
c   Benign prostatic hypertrophy

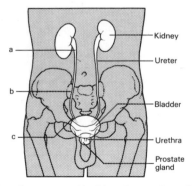

Figure 43. The urinary tract. (a), (b) and (c): points of narrowing of the ureter.

Investigations of the urinary tract

Radiography of the kidneys, ureters and bladder. Radio-opaque stones (about 80% of all urinary tract calculi) can be visualized by straight abdominal X-ray.

Intravenous pyelography. Water-soluble iodine (for example, Hypaque), administered intravenously, is filtered by the glomerulus, taken up in the tubules, concentrated in the urine and excreted. A series of X-rays is taken after the contrast medium has been injected. Disorders which alter the shape of the collecting system, such as dilatation due to obstruction, can be diagnosed.

Angiography. The renal arteries may be cannulated via the femoral artery (see p. 74) and the arterial supply to the kidneys visualized.

Cystoscopy. A rigid scope, with a light source, is introduced through the urethra; the bladder can be visualized and biopsies of the bladder wall taken. A similar instrument is used, with attachments, to resect and cauterize the prostate gland via the urethra.

Retrograde pyelography. Radio-opaque material, such as Hypaque, can be introduced into the ureter by means of a fine catheter through the cystoscope and X-rays taken of the structure of the pelvis, the kidney and the ureter.

Renal biopsy. A needle biopsy of renal tissue can be taken, using a trocar and cannula.

Ultrasound. This may be used to differentiate between a cyst and a renal tumour.

Haematological assays

Blood urea level. This is an indicator of normal kidney function (normal value: 2.5–7.5 mmol/l).

Serum acid phosphatase level. This is increased when there is a carcinoma of the prostate gland.

Serum electrolyte and calcium levels. Electrolyte regulation is a function of the kidney. Serum calcium may be raised in certain metabolic conditions where calculi are present.

Urinalysis

24-hour collection of urine. All the urine voided in a 24-hour period is collected as follows:

Day 1   6 a.m. (for example)   first specimen (discarded)
Day 2   6 a.m. (for example)   last specimen collected

Creatinine clearance test. This is a test of renal efficiency requiring a 24-hour collection of urine. (The normal volume of blood cleared of creatinine in one minute is 70–130 ml.)

Urine examination and analysis. This is a common ward procedure and is invariably a requirement before any surgical procedure. Certain substances are not normally excreted in the urine; if any are present, further investigation is required and this may lead to a diagnosis of another condition, such as diabetes mellitus.

- The presence of blood, ketones, bile, glucose or protein, together with pH of the urine, can be assessed using diagnostic reagent strips (such as Ames Labstix).
- Specific gravity (relative density) is measured relative to water (normal: 1.002–1.040).
- Urine can be examined visually for the presence of blood, pus and foreign bodies such as gravel or stones.
- Bacteria, if present, may be suspected from a characteristic, unpleasant smell. Urine is normally clear, amber in colour and acid (pH 6).

Identification of needs

- Information concerning the reasons for specific preparations for investigations must be given clearly and reinforced where appropriate. It should not be assumed that commonly used medical and nursing jargon will be readily understood, especially when anxiety may already be acting as a barrier to assimilation; for example, does 'nil by mouth' mean 'no fluid' as well as 'no food'?

Related nursing activities

Intravenous pyelography
Faeces or flatus in the colon may obscure the view of the urinary

tract on X-ray, so an aperient is essential before this investigation.

- Patients may be sensitive to the iodine present in the radio-opaque substance administered and should be questioned regarding any known sensitivity. An anaphylactic reaction is possible and precautions should be taken against this (antihistamines and corticosteroids should be available).
- Unpleasant symptoms are sometimes experienced and should be discussed. For example, there may be a burning sensation all over the body, especially the head, and a metallic taste.
- Fluids may be restricted for a short time immediately prior to the procedure, but this will be dependent on the patient's condition and the radiographer's wishes. Mouthwashes should be offered and care taken to prevent the inadvertent offering (or the patient's drinking) of a cup of tea or coffee.

Cystoscopy and retrograde pyelography
- These investigations are usually carried out under a general anaesthetic (see p. 8).
- Mild analgesia may be required after the procedure.
- Bed-rest should be encouraged until the patient is fully recovered from the anaesthetic.
- Fluids should be offered as soon as possible.
- Any urine passed must be observed for the presence of blood (haematuria).
- Retrograde pyelography usually requires the patient to be transported from the operating theatre to an X-ray department; care should be taken to ensure that the catheters are secured against accidental removal.

Renal biopsy
- Sedation is helpful before this procedure is carried out.
- Careful instruction must be given regarding breathing requirements when the trocar is inserted.
- Bed-rest is essential after the procedure.
- Pressure should be applied to the site and it should be regularly observed for bleeding.
- General observation for signs of internal haemorrhage must be undertaken.

Blood specimens

- The patient must be supported through this harmless but often frightening experience.
- The skin must be meticulously cleaned.
- Specimens must be despatched properly labelled and with sufficient information for correct investigation.

Urine collection and analysis

- If urine is to be collected over 24 hours, the most effective way is to give the responsibility for its collection to the patient where appropriate. The patient feels himself involved and contributing to his care; it also serves to occupy his mind over a period of time which may otherwise seem excessively long and empty.
- Urine must be collected in a clean, dry container. If it is for urinalysis on the ward it should not be allowed to stand for any length of time.
- All results must be charted and any abnormality reported. (Inadvertent contamination, for instance menstrual blood in a specimen, can result in a false-positive finding.)
- Collection of a mid-stream specimen is a clean procedure, so discreet, precise and thoughtful advice must be offered and assistance with the procedure given to those who are unable, for reasons such as physical disability, to obtain the specimen themselves.
- Catheter specimens should be obtained from the catheter tubing with a syringe; the closed drainage system should not be broken for this purpose. Asepsis must be maintained throughout.

Urinary tract infection is the commonest cause of hospital-acquired infection, accounting for about 40% of all cases.

Benign prostatic hypertrophy and prostatectomy

The prostate is an encapsulated gland which encircles the base of the male bladder; it consists of two lobes. Hypertrophy (the aetiology of which is unknown) may be present after the age of 50 years; 80% of all males over the age of 80 years are affected. The increase in the size of the gland may obstruct the bladder outlet and a middle lobe may develop and act as a valve, preventing micturition.

Nursing care before prostatectomy

Identification of needs

The patient may have been much troubled by prostatic symptoms for some time and the extent of the symptoms will determine his care preoperatively. There may be:

a dysuria (a burning sensation on micturition) and a poor stream
b frequency or urgency
c nocturia
d dribbling

These symptoms are disconcerting and cause distress to a previously continent person.

Acute retention of urine is sometimes the presenting symptom when other symptoms may have gone unnoticed or unheeded. Catheterization is usually undertaken: it immediately relieves the extreme discomfort which accompanies acute retention. The catheter will be left in place if the prostate gland is found to be enlarged and obstructing the outlet.

Related nursing activities

- Placing the patient in a bed close to a lavatory, together with discreet offers of a change of pyjamas, if necessary, can boost confidence.
- The patient who undergoes prostatectomy is frequently elderly and may not hear or see very well; he will need very careful preparation regarding postoperative events. For example, the reasons for a urethral catheter, irrigation procedures and fluid replacement by infusion should be explained.
- The size of an enlarged prostate gland can be assessed per rectum. (For nursing activities related to this investigation see p. 134.)
- The optimum conditions for prostatectomy are (a) a normal serum urea, (b) sterile urine, and (c) normal renal function.

Investigations required

1 Intravenous pyelography
2 Haematological assay (urea and acid phosphatase), grouping and cross-matching
3 Mid-stream specimen of urine for bacterial culture and antibiotic sensitivity testing.

4 Chest X-ray and electrocardiogram

The nurse is responsible for psychological and social support, advising both patient and relatives of significant time of investigations and results, and also for specific physical preparations such as bowel preparation.

- Acute retention of urine. If the patient is catheterized it is usually considered that a very large amount of urine should not be drained immediately. The tubing may be clamped after a litre has been drained and the residual urine allowed to drain slowly.

Types of prostatectomy

Transurethral prostatectomy (Figure 44a). The cystoscope is inserted per urethra, the prostate gland is removed piecemeal and the site diathermied or frozen. Postoperative drainage is by means of a urethral (Foley type) catheter.

Suprapubic or transvesical prostatectomy (extraperitoneal approach) (Figure 44b). A suprapubic incision is made, the bladder incised and the prostate gland enucleated with the finger, via the bladder neck. Drainage involves a cystotomy drain, suprapubic drainage and a urethral catheter.

Retropubic prostatectomy (extraperitoneal approach) (Figure 44c). Here an approach is made between the pubic bone and the bladder. The capsule of the prostate is incised and the enlarged lobe of the gland enucleated. The bladder is not opened. Drainage is by means of a tube from the site of the prostate and a urethral catheter.

Perineal approach. This is rarely used in Great Britain, but is common in the USA. Drainage is through a tube inserted in the perineum (between scrotum and rectum) and a urethral catheter.

Nursing care after prostatectomy

Identification of needs

- Patients are frequently in the age group in which other pathology such as cardiac or pulmonary disease may be present; the patient may be hypoxic and confused after an

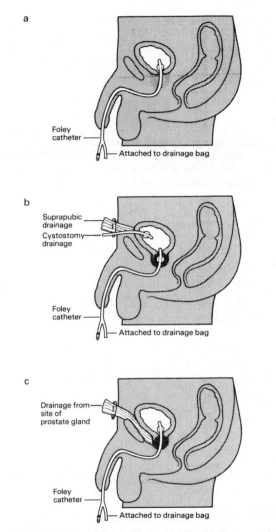

Figure 44. Types of prostatectomy, showing drainage employed: (a) transurethral prostatectomy; (b) suprapubic (transvesical) prostatectomy (extraperitoneal approach); (c) retropubic prostatectomy (extraperitoneal approach).

anaesthetic. A safe environment must be ensured, particularly during the first postoperative night, when the presence of a catheter may be experienced as a desire to pass urine. The urethral catheter should not be pinned to the bed linen, but may sometimes be strapped to the anterior aspect of the upper leg.
- The urine outlet must be unobstructed.

Related nursing activities
- Clot formation must not be permitted to obstruct the flow of urine through the urethra, so a closed system of bladder irrigation is used. Urine will be bloodstained initially, but will become clear in about 24–48 hours; bladder irrigation will continue until this is achieved. If urine flow appears obstructed this should be reported; the bladder may become grossly distended and eventually rupture if this problem is left unattended.
- Analgesia commensurate with the patient's age and general condition should be administered.
- Intravenous infusion may be in progress until free oral fluid intake is established.
- A fluid input/output chart is of vital importance, to record return of irrigation fluid, urine output and commensurate intake.

Continuing care
- Urethral catheter care. Some surgeons request slight traction on the catheter; this can be achieved by appropriate taping to the anterior aspect of the thigh. It is desirable for the legs to be free of pyjama trousers to promote drainage through the tubing by gravity. A knee-length cotton gown will preserve the dignity of the individual and facilitate drainage.
- The drainage bag should be emptied as an aseptic procedure and never allowed to rest on the floor. The bag must be attached to a hanger designed for this purpose.
- Regular and careful cleaning of the urethral meatus should be carried out.
- The catheter will be removed between the fourth and seventh day when haematuria is no longer present. A specimen of urine will be obtained before removal of the catheter for microbiological assay. After catheter removal some problems may become apparent, for example:

a No urine is passed and the bladder is palpable. The catheter may need to be reinserted by a doctor; this may be a difficult procedure if the cause of retention is oedema of the urethra.

b The patient has an irresistible desire to pass small but frequent amounts of urine or is incontinent. This will be a difficult time for a patient who may think that a symptom he had before the surgical procedure has not been alleviated. Invariably continence will eventually be achieved and he should be encouraged to increase the time between each micturition until this is achieved. A mid-stream specimen of urine will be obtained for culture, as a urinary tract infection may be the cause of persistent frequency and dysuria.

c Constipation. This should be relieved by oral aperients, sufficient fluids and foods high in dietary fibre.

- A suprapubic catheter incision (for cystotomy drainage) should be kept clean and dry—it is often the site of a wound infection; there may be some urine leakage at this site when the catheter is removed.
- There should be no urine drainage from the bed of the prostate gland (after retropubic prostatectomy); dressings should be carefully observed when renewed.

A late complication of prostatectomy may be urethral stricture; this will require dilatation under general anaesthesia.

Carcinoma of the prostate gland

Prostatic carcinoma may metastasize via the pelvic bones and vertebrae. Treatment may be by radical prostatectomy, involving removal of the prostate gland, a portion of the bladder and lymph nodes. Radiotherapy may decrease the size of a tumour. The female hormone oestrogen will control the growth of metastases. Alternatively a transurethral resection of the prostate gland may be performed, and may be followed by oestrogen administration.

Bladder surgery

Papillomas are wart-like growths of the bladder wall; they are benign but predispose to malignancy. They are treated by diathermy, followed-up by regular check cystoscopy and biopsy.

Malignant bladder tumour is treated by partial cystectomy if the base of the bladder is not involved. If total bladder removal (total cystectomy) is undertaken a urinary diversion will be necessary. In this procedure a loop of terminal ileum is isolated with a portion of mesentery and its blood supply intact. The proximal end of this portion of ileum is closed, the ureters are implanted into its wall, and the distal end is brought to the surface as a urine-excreting stoma; this segment of the ileum acts as a passage for urine—an ileal conduit. When the loop has been isolated, the remainder of the ileum is anastomosed, re-establishing continuity of the tract.

Alternative surgical procedures involve implanting the ureters into the colon or rectum, which will act as an alternative reservoir for urine.

Nursing care of the patient undergoing total cystectomy

Identification of needs–preoperative

- This surgery brings about a radical alteration in body image, which needs carefully planned preoperative preparation (see p. 131).
- The operation to be undertaken is extensive and the patient needs to be physically ready, that is well nourished and well rested.

Related nursing activities–preoperative

- As for gastrointestinal surgical procedures bowel preparation is important. The aim is a clean, empty bowel and preparation will be according to the surgeon's wishes and ward practice.

Identification of needs–postoperative

- Continuing psychological support, information and advice is needed in order to achieve maximum physical potential and social rehabilitation for the patient.

Related nursing activities–postoperative

- For urinary stoma care see p. 130. The colour of the 'spout' is of paramount importance as an indicator of an adequate blood supply to the conduit; any changes must be reported immediately.
- Careful, close observation must be made for early signs of peritonitis (see p. 114), for any significant deterioration in

urinary output, and for indications of electrolyte imbalance, such as the patient becoming weak, confused and lethargic.

● Scrupulous attention must be given to drainage tubing; surrounding skin must be kept clean and dry.

● When the patient has made some physical recovery, the psychological aspects of the radical alteration of body image will be of primary significance and advice regarding management of the stoma when he returns home should be introduced when it will most effectively be assimilated.

Calculi (renal stones)

The operation 'to cut for the stone' *(lithotomy)* was described as early as the beginning of the 18th century. A large percentage of stones are formed from calcium, some from uric acid and others are a mixture of crystalline substances.

A stone may form anywhere within the urinary tract; formation within the calyces of the kidney produces a staghorn calculus, a stone which takes on the shape of that portion of the kidney. There are three points at which the ureter narrows (Figure 43); a stone which forms or lodges in the ureter may cause extreme pain (renal colic) as the ureter actively attempts to overcome the obstruction. The pain may be experienced in the loin area, radiating to the scrotum in the male and the labia in the female.

Nursing activities related to the patient with acute renal colic

● Strong analgesia should be administered, for example intramuscular pethidine 100 mg every four hours or any other drug, as ordered, which will be effective for the relief of this agonizing pain. An antiemetic may also be prescribed since the patient with renal colic may be nauseated and vomiting.

● Bedclothes and pillows should be arranged comfortably: the patient is often restless, hot, sweaty and very anxious.

● As much fluid should be offered orally as can reasonably be tolerated, in order to increase production of urine and possible flushing of the stone from the narrow ureter.

● Careful observation should be made of all urine passed; it should be strained to detect the presence of gravel or stones. Any stone passed may be analysed and the result of this analysis together with haematological assay may determine future treatment.

- A calcium-restricted diet may be necessary; careful explanation and the preparation of a specific diet sheet will help the patient adhere to the restrictions.
- A fluid balance chart should be maintained and urine should be tested for the presence of blood, as the passage of a stone may traumatize the urethra.
- Further metabolic investigations may be required to determine the origins of the problem.

Surgery for removal of stone

1 Nephrolithotomy: removal of stone from the body of the kidney.
2 Pyelolithotomy: removal of stone from the renal pelvis.
3 Ureterolithotomy: removal of stone from the ureter.

If the stone is contained within the lower third of the ureter, an instrument (the Dormier basket) may be inserted via the cystoscope and the stone removed. A stone within the upper two-thirds of the ureter, the pelvis or the kidney substance will be removed through an upper abdominal loin incision.

4 Suprapubic cystotomy—removal of stone from the bladder.

Related nursing activities
- A drainage tube is always inserted to prevent leakage of urine into surrounding tissues; it will be removed when drainage is minimal or has ceased, according to the surgeon's wishes.

Removal of a kidney (nephrectomy)

Reasons for the removal of a kidney include: severe trauma, polycystic kidney, and malignancy.

Identification of needs
Before the operation the patient's ability to understand information regarding kidney function must be carefully assessed, before existing knowledge can be built on, extended and reinforced where appropriate. The body's ability to adapt and function adequately with only one kidney may be difficult to comprehend, but it is an essential factor to impart when helping

the patient to overcome the surgical intervention and its aftermath.

Related nursing activities–preoperative
- Information should be given about the drainage tube which will be inserted to drain the site from which the kidney has been removed.
- Severe discomfort may be experienced postoperatively; the possible reasons for the pain and the means available for its effective relief should be discussed.
- If the surgeon has raised the possibility of radiotherapy after the surgical procedure, this course of treatment may need further careful explanation. The patient should be allowed to express the fears and anxiety which are easily aroused when this subject is first mentioned. Raised anxiety levels can obstruct the accurate assimilation of information.

Related nursing activities–postoperative
- Positioning. The aim should be a comfortable, well supported position which allows the patient to make minor adjustments as he desires, but the drainage tube must be protected from occlusion at all times.
- Observation of drainage. Any sudden excessive drainage must be reported at once. A slipped ligature can result in a severe and rapid drop in circulating blood volume.
- Fluid balance. Oral fluids must be encouraged as soon as the patient is able to tolerate them (i.e., when bowel sounds are present and there is no abdominal distension). The urine output must be measured and recorded. A catheter is not normally introduced after this surgical procedure.
- Analgesia. Pain must never be allowed to become oppressive.

Future health considerations
- The patient should be counselled to adopt a careful but not restrictive lifestyle, avoiding situations with high risks of infection, for example large gatherings of people. Whilst he may be active in sport, some activities may be hazardous if the possibility of physical injury should endanger his remaining kidney.
- Medication should only be taken if prescribed by a clinician who is aware that he has had a kidney removed.

Further reading

Horsley, J.A. (Michigan Nurses Association: CURN Project) (1981) *Closed Urinary Drainage Systems.* (Using Research to Improve Nursing Practice Series) New York: Grune & Stratton.

Appendix

SI UNITS

Basic units

Physical quantity	Name of unit	Symbol
Mass	kilogram	kg
Length	metre	m
Time	second	s
Electric current	Ampere	A
Temperature	kelvin	K
Luminous intensity	candela	cd
Amount of substance	mole	mol

Prefixes used for multiples

Figure	Prefix	Sign
10^{-12}	pico	p
10^{-9}	nano	n
10^{-6}	micro	μ
10^{-3}	milli	m
10^{-2}	centi	c
10^{-1}	deci	d
10	deca	da
10^{2}	hecto	h
10^{3}	kilo	k
10^{6}	mega	M
10^{9}	giga	G
10^{12}	tera	T

Weights

1000 micrograms (μg) = 1 milligram
1000 milligrams (mg) = 1 gram
1000 grams (g)   = 1 kilogramme
1000 kilograms (kg) = 1 metric tonne

Capacity

1000 microlitres (μl) = 1 millilitre (ml)
  10 millilitres   = 1 centilitre (cl)
 100 millilitres   = 10 centilitres = 1 decilitre (dl)
1000 millilitres   = 100 centilitres =10 decilitres =
                        1 litre (l)

  1 cubic centimetre (cm³ *or* cc) = 1 millilitre
  1 cubic decimetre (dm³)   = 1 litre

Domestic equivalents (approximate)
1 teaspoon   =   5 ml
1 dessertspoon =   10 ml
1 tablespoon   =   20 ml
1 sherryglass =   60 ml
1 teacup   = 142 ml
1 breakfastcup = 230 ml
1 tumbler   = 285 ml

ENERGY

A dietetic Calorie is the amount of heat required to raise the temperature of 1 litre of water 1°C and is equal to 4.184 kilojoules.

1 gram of fat will produce 38 kilojoules or 9 Calories.
1 gram of protein will produce 17 kilojoules or 4 Calories.
1 gram of carbohydrate will produce 17 kilojoules or 4 Calories.

WEIGHTS AND HEIGHTS

Average weight and height of children and young people

Boys			Girls	
Weight (kg)	Height (cm)	Age	Weight (kg)	Height (cm)
3.4	50.6	Birth	3.36	50.2
10.07	75.2	1 year	9.75	74.2
12.56	87.5	2 years	12.29	86.6
14.61	96.2	3 years	14.42	95.7
16.51	103.4	4 years	16.42	103.2
18.89	110.0	5 years	18.58	109.4
21.91	117.5	6 years	21.09	115.9
24.54	124.1	7 years	23.68	122.3
27.26	130.0	8 years	26.35	128.0
29.94	135.5	9 years	28.94	132.9
32.61	140.3	10 years	31.89	138.6
35.2	144.2	11 years	35.74	144.7
38.28	146.6	12 years	39.74	151.9
42.18	155.0	13 years	44.95	157.1
48.81	162.7	14 years	49.17	159.6
54.48	167.8	15 years	51.48	161.1
58.83	171.6	16 years	53.07	162.2
61.78	172.7	17 years	54.02	162.5
63.05	174.5	18 years	54.39	162.5

Average weight of adults aged 30

Height (cm)	Weight (kg)		
	Small build	Medium build	Large build
Women			
152.5	48.5	53.9	60.7
157.5	51.2	56.6	63.9
162.5	53.9	59.8	67.5
167.5	57.1	63.4	71.6
172.5	60.2	67.0	75.7
178.0	63.4	70.2	78.9
Men			
167.5	58.4	64.8	72.9
172.5	61.6	68.4	77.0
177.5	65.7	72.9	82.0
183	70.7	78.4	87.9
188	75.7	83.8	94.2

NORMAL VALUES

	SI units	Old units
Blood		
Activated partial thromboplastin time	28–35 s	28–35 s
Bleeding time	1–6 min	1–6 min
Clotting time	5–11 min	5–11 min
Haemoglobin	12–18 g/dl	12–18 g/100 ml
Packed cell volume (haematocrit)	0.42–0.50 l/l	42–50 mg/100 ml
pH	7.35–7.45	7.35–7.45
Pco_2	5–6 kPa	38–45 mmHg
Po_2	11–15 kPa	80–110 mmHg
Platelets	$150–400 \times 10^9$/litre	150 000– 400 000 mm^3
Prothrombin time	10–14 s	10–14 s
Red cells	$4–6 \times 10^{12}$/litre	4 million– 6 million/mm^3
Sedimentation rate		
men	0–5 mm	0–5 mm
women	0–7 mm	0–7 mm
White cells	$4–11 \times 10^9$/litre	$4–11 \times 10^9$/litre

NORMAL VALUES—*(continued)*

	SI units	Old units
Plasma		
Bicarbonate	21–28 mmol/litre	21–28 mEq/litre
Chloride	98–107 mmol/litre	98–107 mEq/litre
Fibrinogen	1.5–4.0 g/litre	1.5–4.0 g/litre
Glucose (fasting)	2.5–4.7 mmol/litre	45–80 mg/100 ml
Potassium	3.5–5.0 mmol/litre	3.5–5.0 mEq/litre
Sodium	135–145 mmol/litre	135–145 mEq/litre
Urea	3–7 mmol/litre	20–40 mg/100 ml
Urine		
Creatinine	10.0–15.0 mmol/ 24 h	1.1–1.7 g/24 h
Urea	170–580 mmol/litre	1.0–3.5 g/100 ml
Relative density (specific gravity)	1.002–1.040	1002–1040
CSF		
Glucose	2.8–3.9 mmol/litre	45–70 mg/100 ml
Protein	150–300 mg/litre	15–30 mg/100 ml
Thyroid function tests		
Total serum thyroxine	58–128 nmol/litre	
Free binding capacity	90–105%	
Free thyroxine index	53–142	
Serum T_3	1.5–3.5 nmol/litre	
Thyroid-stimulating hormone (TSH)	1–5 mU/litre	

Index